health
& beauty

ACKNOWLEDGEMENTS

I would like to thank Catie Ziller and Anne Wilson for making everything happen, and Jackie Frank and Matt Handbury for their support and the opportunity to do this book. I'd also like to thank Sara Beaney for her enthusiasm, ongoing support and outstanding creativity, and Greg Delves for his innovative photography and inspiration – I couldn't have done it without you both. Special thanks to Annette McKenzie for her make-up and Kevin Murphy for all his hairdos, to Jacquie Brown for her endless hours of hard work and to Rowena Lennox for her attention to detail. To Brendan, Nick and Sarah for keeping me sane and all my family and friends for believing in me.

Special thanks to Vicci Bentley for compiling the Alternative Therapy guide; Tania Cusack for the spa menus; beauty therapist Catriona Clayton; naturopath Lucy Sharman at Hilton Lifestream; Dr John de Launey; Julie Gundlach, clinical aromatherapist, Swedish massage therapist and reflexologist; and Joanna McKenzie, remedial massage therapist at Zen: The Art of Body Maintenance; Anna Marchant; Anna Barr; and interiors stylist Sibella Court. Thank you for the loan of props and clothes from Aero, Space, Orson Blake, Calvin Klein, Blackmores, Clinique, Estee Lauder, Issey Myake, Shu Uemura, C Design, Jaclin Chouchana and Gucci.

This edition published 2005 by Igloo Books Ltd,

Henson Way, Telford Way Industrial Estate,

Kettering, Northants, NN16 8PX.

info@igloo-books.com.

Copyright © Murdoch Books Pty Limited

www.murdochbooks.com.au

Art Director/Designer: Sara Beaney, Photographer: Greg Delves, Stylist: Jane Campsie
Make-up: Annette McKenzie using make-up from The Look by Napoleon, Hair: Kevin Murphy and Campbell McAuley
Models: Lucia and Carolyn Ranicar, Editor: Jacquie Brown

ISBN: 1-84561-114-4

This book contains information on a wide range of health and beauty topics. It is not intended as a medical reference book, but as a source of information. Readers are not advised to attempt self-treatment (especially using essential oils) if pregnant or suffering from serious or long-term problems without consulting a qualified expert. Neither the author or the publisher can be held responsible for any adverse reaction to the recommendations and instructions contained within this book.

health
& beauty

JANE CAMPSIE

igloo

PHILOSOPHY

health and beauty is an authoritative guide that addresses the strains of modern living, focusing on the link between your inner health and outer beauty. Today, health and beauty is not about faddish diets, whimsical trends, or trying to change who you are. It is about being happy with the way you look and feel. You don't need supermodel looks or a wafer-thin physique to look good. The modern approach to beauty is to make the most of your natural assets and focus on your positive traits. It's about subtle enhancement, not drastic transformation. The aim is to improve your self-image and self-esteem.

In the initial stages of planning this book, we decided to focus on a realistic approach to health and beauty. I have searched to find solutions to everyday health and beauty problems. This book shows you how to monitor your body's health requirements, to perfect make-up application, to master the art of aromatherapy and teaches you self-massage. It encompasses a complete way of life to improve the way you look and feel.

Use this book to devise a regime to suit you and make health and beauty an integral part of your lifestyle – assess your diet, take time out and indulge yourself with pampering treatments, look at enjoyable recreational activities to keep you fit and focus on your inner health.

I hope you find this book easy to follow, reap the benefits and enjoy it as much as I have enjoyed writing it.

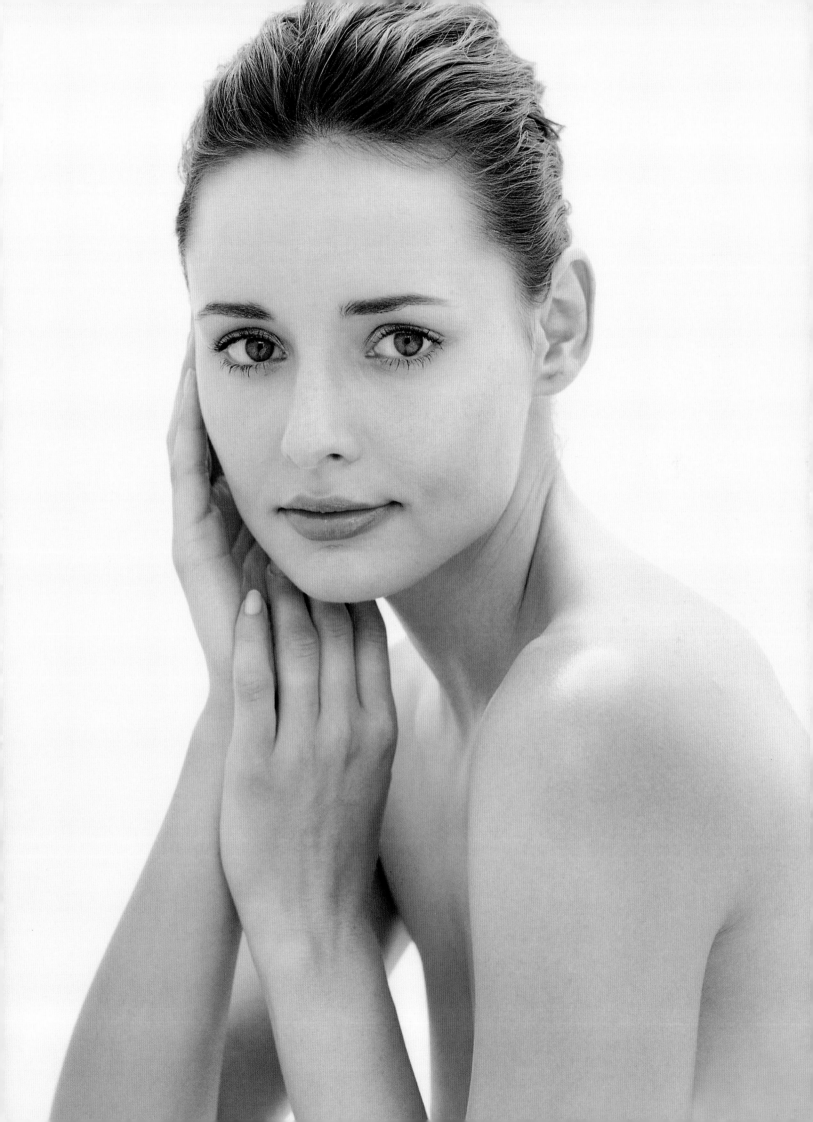

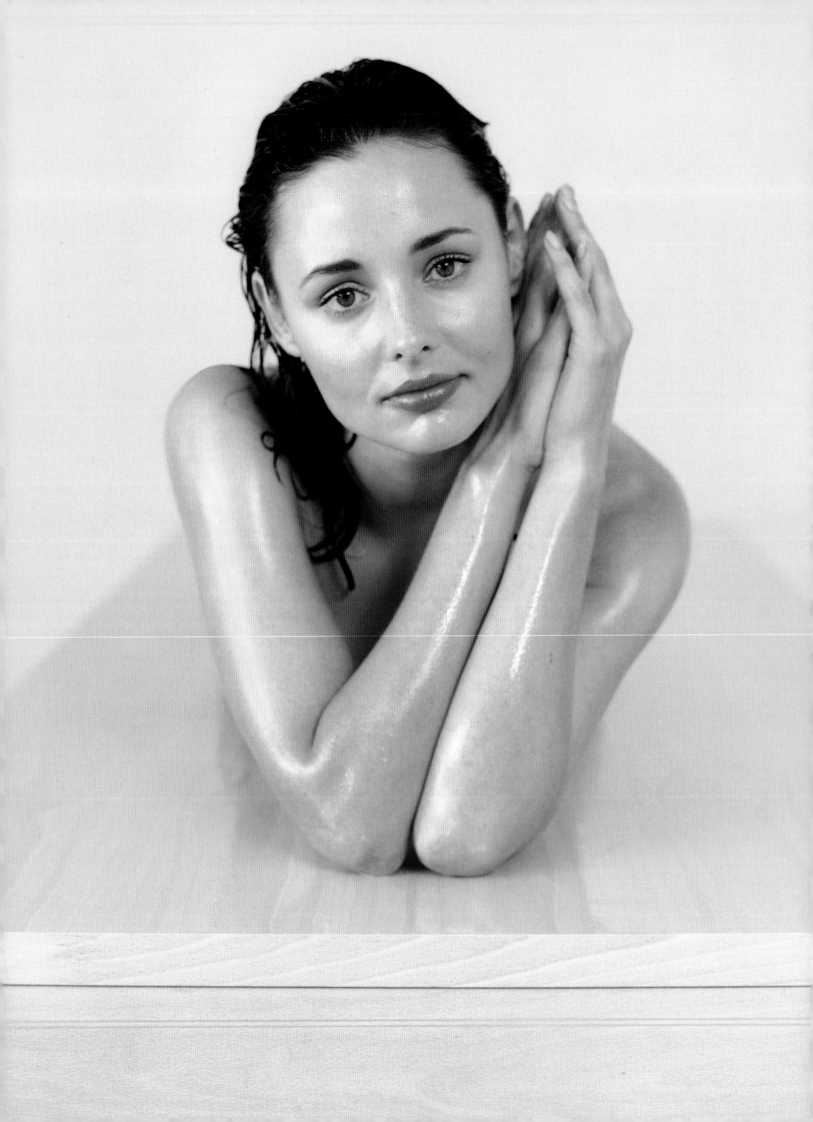

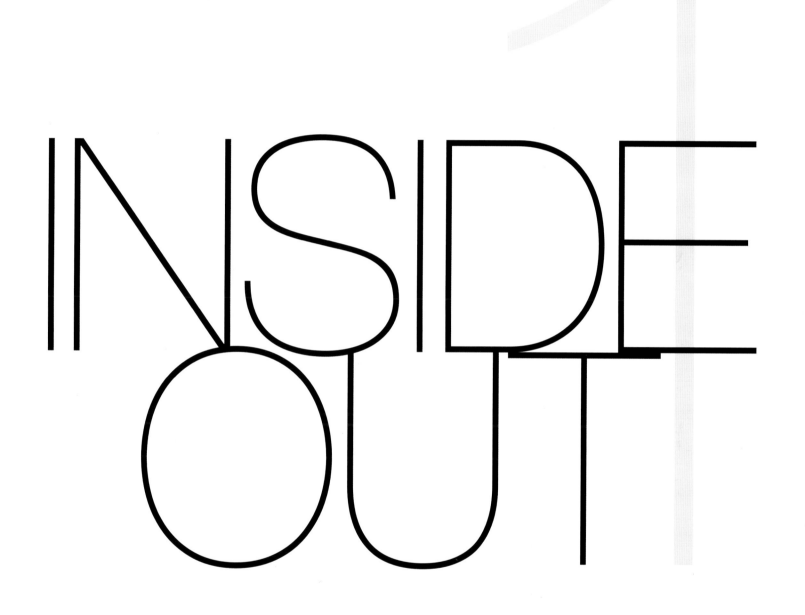

INSIDE OUT

INNER HEALTH AFFECTS OUTER BEAUTY. TO ADDRESS YOUR BODY'S NEEDS, FOLLOW A NUTRITIONAL CLEANSING REGIME. IT WILL BENEFIT THE WAY YOU LOOK AND IMPROVE THE WAY YOU FEEL.

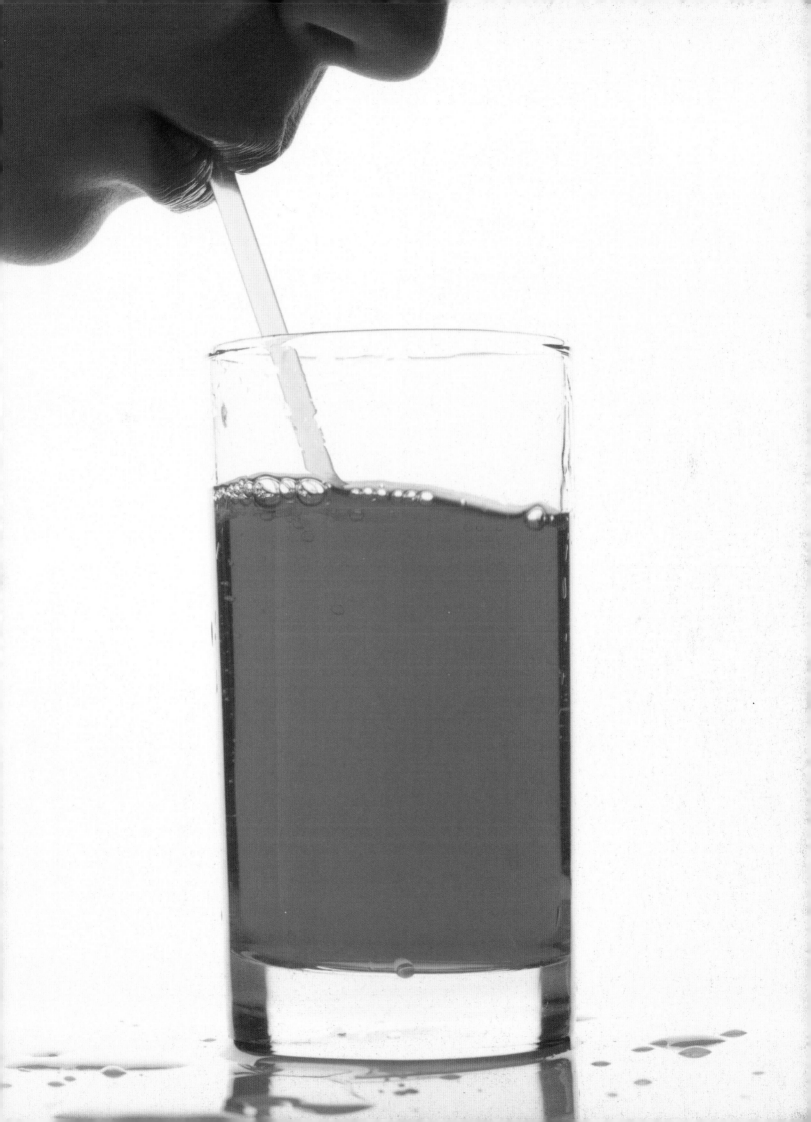

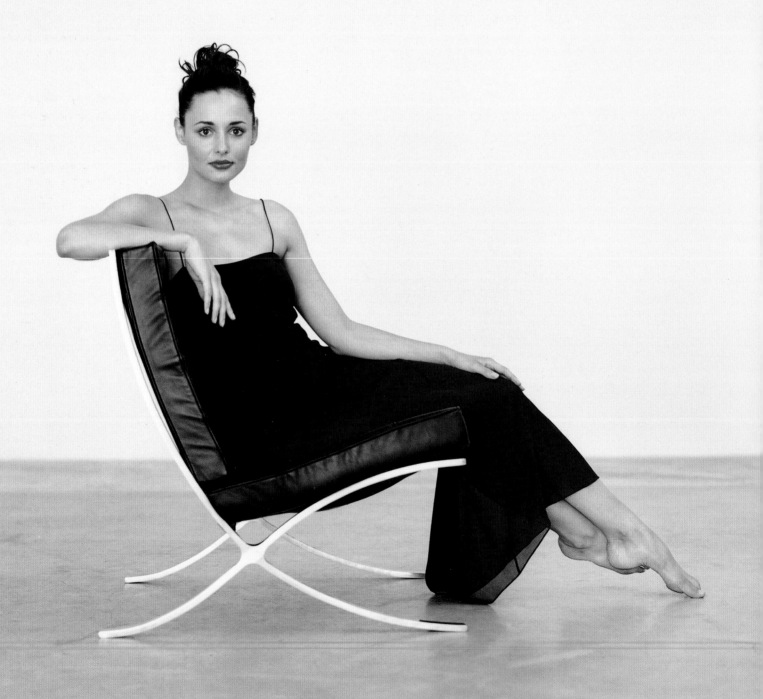

INNER HEALTH

Does your skin look dull and lifeless? Do you wake up in the morning feeling tired and 'hung-over,' even though you haven't been drinking the night before? If so, it's time to cancel out the detrimental effects of modern living and treat your body to a complete cleansing regime.

THE BY-PRODUCTS OF SMOKING, processed foods, late nights, alcohol and stressful, sedentary lifestyles take their toll on the body. They put extra strain on the organs (especially the liver) and use up or destroy vital nutrients, which can lead to conditions ranging from skin problems and allergies to fatigue, premature ageing and more serious diseases such as cancer. As all of this activity occurs internally, an overload of toxins can often go undetected. The most common symptoms are nausea, headaches or recurrent skin complaints.

BODY CLEANSING

The most effective way to 'spring-clean' your body is to follow a raw fruit and vegetable fast. In addition to detoxifying your system and flushing out your colon, it will improve your energy levels, increase your ability to concentrate and perhaps even enhance your outlook on life.

FRUITS AND VEGETABLES contain specific nutrients and compounds called phytochemicals. These are powerful substances that help to ward off premature ageing and the development of degenerative diseases. Eliminating other foods temporarily from your diet will take the pressure off your body and stimulate the liver's excretion process.

EMBARK ON A DETOXIFICATION REGIME on the weekend or when your schedule is not too demanding, as you may experience fatigue, headaches, aching muscles, unsettled emotions, diarrhoea, tiredness or skin breakouts. (These are all encouraging signs that your body is detoxifying.) Because of these dramatic changes, eat small meals or drink juice regularly (preferably every 2–3 hours) to ensure that your body's blood-sugar levels remain constant.

NEVER FOLLOW THIS TYPE OF REGIME if you are pregnant, diabetic, epileptic, anaemic or suffering from a serious illness. Aim to incorporate a one-day detox into your lifestyle on a regular basis. For a longer, more intensive detoxification regime, always consult a naturopath for guidance.

HEALTHY SOLUTIONS

To aid digestion and cleanse your palate, start the day with a cup of boiling water mixed with the juice of half a lemon.

To supplement a detox regime, naturopaths recommend taking milk thistle or dandelion, and a good multivitamin and vitamin B complex.

Dry skin brushing while you detox will increase the elimination of wastes from your body.

Invest in a juicer. A blender is not an effective alternative if you want to make a range of fruit and vegetable juices.

Sip juices slowly. This enables the juice to mix with saliva as you drink, enhancing digestion.

Drinking water helps to flush toxins from your body. Aim to drink at least one litre of filtered or bottled spring water daily.

DETOXIFICATION REGIME

The day before starting a fruit and vegetable detox, eat cooked and raw vegetables, brown rice and salads. Avoid animal products, alcohol and sweetened foods. Wean yourself off caffeine by substituting tea and coffee with herbal teas.

ON YOUR FASTING DAY, consume raw fruit and vegetables such as apples, pineapples, mangoes, pawpaws, watermelon, grapes, pears, celery, carrots, tomatoes, spinach and beetroot. Vary the way you prepare your chosen foods: juices are easy for your body to assimilate quickly and efficiently, taking on average only 10–15 minutes to digest, but eating fruit and vegetables in their natural state is essential for roughage.

TRY THE FOLLOWING MENU PLAN during your detoxification regime: for breakfast, have a large glass of fresh juice made from apples, grapes, oranges, and grapefruit blended with a green leafy vegetable. Have a serving of fresh fruit and drink herbal tea sweetened with honey. For lunch, drink fresh vegetable juices (choose from spinach, celery, carrot, tomato, raw beetroot or mixed vegetable) and have a large salad. For dinner, have a glass of vegetable or fruit juice and a light salad. Drink herbal tea or coffee substitutes.

JUICING REMEDIES

Address common ailments with fresh fruits and raw vegetables. If you suffer from constipation, try drinking the juice of fruit and vegetables that have a natural laxative effect, such as rhubarb, apples, spinach, prunes and pears.

IF YOU SUFFER FROM WATER RETENTION, increase your intake of potassium-rich foods such as bananas, prunes, raisins, figs, seaweed, broccoli, spinach, fish, green vegetables, celery and apples. Juices made from watermelon, grape and cucumber will also help to eliminate excess water from your system.

IF YOU SUFFER FROM ECZEMA, increase your intake of foods rich in bioflavonoids, such as sweet peppers, tomatoes, parsley, and cabbage, to help reduce surface inflammation. Eating foods containing zinc, such as carrots, garlic and ginger, and essential fatty acids, such as fish, nuts and seeds, will benefit eczema.

IF YOU SUFFER FROM PRE-MENSTRUAL SYNDROME (PMS), opt for juices made from pineapple. This fruit contains an enzyme called bromelain, which has a soothing, relaxing effect on the body's muscle tissue. It also helps to ease period pain.

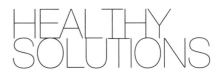

HEALTHY SOLUTIONS

Spice up raw juices with ginger. You don't need to peel it, just cut it into small slices before juicing.

For effective body cleansing drink fruit juices in the morning and savoury vegetable juices during the rest of the day.

After your cleansing regime, don't be tempted to feast on unhealthy foods – it will undo all of the good work. Continue eating fruit, salads, vegetables and vegetable soups, and then gradually introduce wholefoods and solids to maintain a balanced diet.

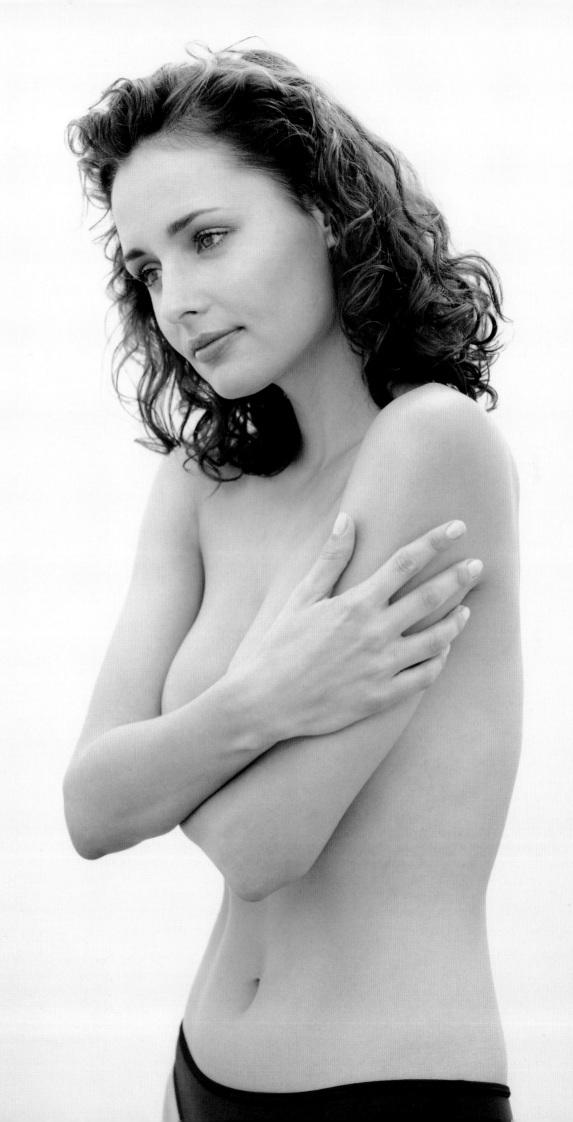

NUTRITIONAL BENEFITS

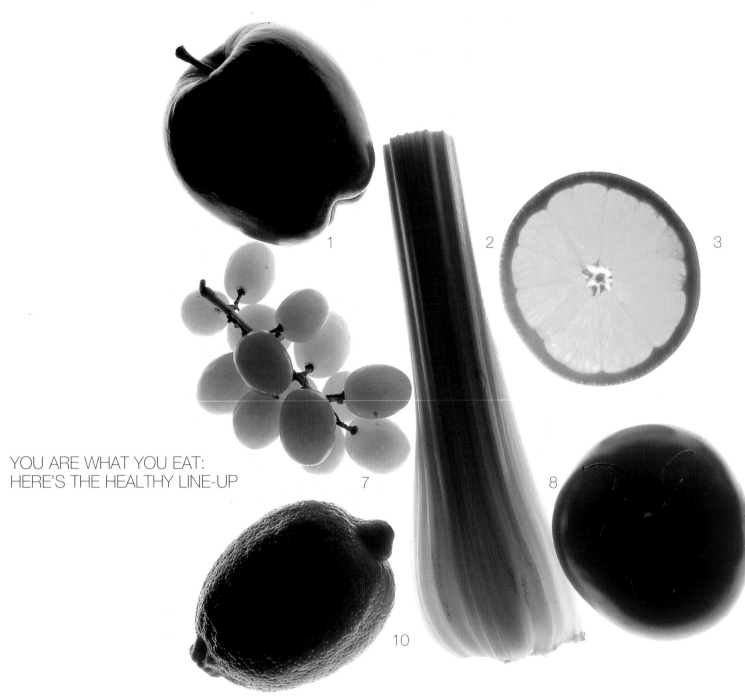

YOU ARE WHAT YOU EAT:
HERE'S THE HEALTHY LINE-UP

1 APPLE contains beta-carotene, vitamins B and C and potassium, and is a great source of fibre. Apples don't need to be peeled or cored for juicing and are ideal to blend with most other fruits and vegetables. 2 CELERY benefits the complexion and maintains healthy blood. For a nutritious, tasty juice, blend celery with carrot and apple. 3 ORANGE (like other citrus fruits) is loaded with vitamin C and is an excellent energy booster. Always peel oranges before juicing – the skins of all citrus fruits are waxed to preserve their shelf life. 4 BEETROOT is an extremely effective blood and kidney cleanser. As a juice, it can be combined with other vegetables such as celery, carrots, spinach and cucumber. Wash the leafy tops of the beetroot and include them in the juice. 5 PINEAPPLE contains the enzyme bromelain, which breaks down protein. It is believed to assist in sinus decongestion,

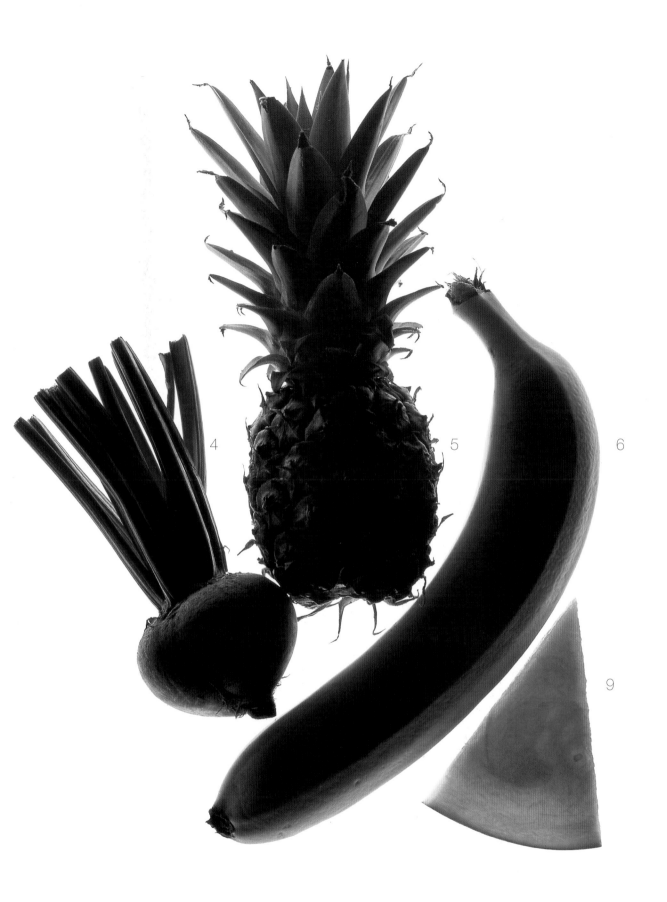

4   5   6

9

to help treat urinary infections, to assist with sleeping problems and is also used as an anti-inflammatory treatment for arthritis. 6 BANANAS are a rich source of potassium, an essential mineral for muscle and nerve functioning. Avoid unripe bananas – they can cause intestinal wind. 7 GRAPES are an excellent source of potassium, and red and black grapes contain vital antioxidants. If you can't sleep, drink juice made from grape and pineapple before going to bed. 8 TOMATO is a useful source of vitamins C and E. (Recurrent mouth ulcers and eczema could be an indication that tomatoes don't agree with you.) 9 WATERMELON contains a high water content that is believed to stimulate the functioning of the kidneys. 10 LEMON is a good palate and liver cleanser, but should be used sparingly because of its high acidity. Don't add more than half a lemon or lime to a glass of juice.

ALTERNATIVE THERAPIES

FINE-TUNE YOUR HEALTH WITH A HOLISTIC APPROACH

AYURVEDIC MEDICINE

Ayurvedic medicine balances general health, controls stress and treats specific complaints that fail to respond to orthodox medicine. This traditional Indian medicine and philosophy system embraces all aspects of well-being and works on the principle that it is possible to live for 100 years, hence its reputation as an anti-ageing system. The human body is governed by three *doshas*, or bio-energies. *Vata* is responsible for movement; *pitta*, metabolism; and *kapha*, growth and structure. Ideally, all *doshas* should be balanced (disharmony can lead to illness). Diet, exercise (especially yoga), massage, meditation and strict lifestyle guidelines all help to maintain this balance. Herbs may be prescribed for specific illnesses.

BUSH FLOWER REMEDIES

Bush flower remedies treat emotions (such as anger, grief, and low self-esteem) that trigger physical conditions. They were devised in the 1930s by English pathologist and bacteriologist Edward Bach, who believed that if plants were floated in pure water in full sunlight, they would energise the water with their molecular imprint. This principle led to the development of over 70 Australian bush flower essences. These include Waratah, which boosts strength and resourcefulness and is used as an anti-stress remedy; and Billy Goat Plum, which dispels self-loathing and encourages sexual fulfilment. Bush flower remedies can be smoothed on the skin in a cream or taken as drops on the tongue.

CRANIO-SACRAL THERAPY

Cranio-sacral therapy treats headaches, migraine, sinus problems, stress, and posture-related shoulder and back pain. It is an offshoot of cranial osteopathy, which uses subtle manipulation to free tension between the bones of the head and spine. The region from the cranium (top of the head) to the sacrum (base of spine) has an energy system with its own subtle pulse. Tension blocks can affect the entire body. Cranio-sacral therapy supports the head, spine and other regions to allow tension to uncoil naturally and the body's energy to flow in the direction it wants to. It involves no pulling, rubbing or massage, just a deeply reassuring sensation of being held gently while your body relaxes.

DANCE THERAPY

Dance therapy, which promotes body awareness, relieves stress, increases mobility and boosts self-esteem, is based on the premise that movement is an important means of non-verbal communication. Dance therapy systems including Laban Dance Therapy and the Chilean 'Biodanza' are useful adjuncts to counselling, psychotherapy and physiotherapy. Sessions are held in groups and can initially be quite confrontational. You are encouraged to describe your feelings through movements to various musical beats. Therapists believe that as you eventually learn to open up, your confidence increases and social interaction becomes easier. The aim is to use your entire body to its full potential.

ELECTRO-CRYSTAL THERAPY

Electro-crystal therapy balances physical and emotional energy, which helps to heal injuries. Devised by English ex-science teacher Harry Oldfield, this controversial system aims to re-tune the body's natural vibrations with electromagnetic fields that are amplified by crystals. An X-ray-like camera scans the body for high-frequency lightwaves that indicate states of energy flow. These are then relayed to a computer screen for diagnosis. The electro-crystal therapist studies the swirling areas of colour for the blocked or weak energy zones underlying the patient's problems. Then electro-magnetic fields are beamed at trouble spots to rebalance the body's energies.

FELDENKRAIS METHOD

This method improves posture and mobility, overcoming stiffness, injury or disability. Devised in the 1940s by ex-atomic physicist, Moshe Feldenkrais, it involves the teaching of gentle movement sequences that optimise and balance posture and movement. The theory of body awareness through movement is taught verbally in classes. Then functional integration is taught on a one-to-one basis, where the teacher guides the pupil through a series of gentle manipulations and touches. Often the process of re-learning freedom of movement begins with slow, strain-free floor exercises that resemble the way babies first stretch and move. The more relaxed a pupil becomes, the freer the movements will be.

GEM THERAPY

Gem therapy balances energies, dispels negatively charged atmospheres and encourages positive thought. The idea that semi-precious and precious stones can be used to heal is thousands of years old. Chosen according to colour and clarity or opaqueness, there is a stone that relates to virtually every human condition. Quartz and amethyst crystals, for example, are both considered universal 'cure-alls' that can also amplify other healing methods. The gems are either placed on or around the body. Some give out energy, while others are thought to absorb pain. They can also be used to channel energy. Wearing gems as protective talismans next to the skin is the most popular form of gem therapy.

HELLERWORK TECHNIQUE

Hellerwork improves posture and mobility, releases emotions, eases injuries and promotes personal growth. Developed by Joseph Heller, who believed that psycho-logical trauma is held in the muscles and fascia (tissues that envelop them), Hellerwork involves deep-reaching restructuring and rebalancing bodywork. Poor posture, for example, may result from low self-esteem, charac-terised by hunched shoulders. Hellerwork concentrates on de-hunching the body and freeing the negative emotions. It entails manipulation ranging from firm to almost invasive. Each session concentrates on a different body zone and the emotion it carries. The release enables both physical and emotional progression.

IRIDOLOGY ANALYSIS

Iridology is a diagnostic method that identifies physical and emotional disorders by analysing the irides, or irises, of the eyes. Iridologists claim that the entire body is reflected by the eyes, because this is where the entire nervous system surfaces. Colour and texture of the iris indicates the patient's state of health and personality type, which may predispose them to illness. (Both present and past problems may be evident.) Various flecks and marks on the eye indicate problems in the relevant body zone. As iridology is diagnostic only, the patient may be referred to a nutritionist or naturopath for treatment. Iridology is also used to monitor orthodox treatments, or to check up on general health.

KINESIOLOGY TREATMENT

Kinesiology treats problems (such as psoriasis, candida, PMS, allergies and bronchitis) that seem to defy other therapies. It is a system of diagnosis and treatment based on muscle testing and works on the principal that the body knows exactly what it needs. The kinesiologist asks a series of health-related questions and applies light, tapping pressures to each arm. If the answer is yes, the arm stays still. If the answer is no, the muscle weakens and the arm drops. As well as diagnosing, tapping can also rid the body of intolerances and allergies. Other energising and clearing techniques involve crystals, essential oils, magnets and homeopathic remedies, which are held against the body during treatment.

LIGHT THERAPY

Light therapy treats depression, stiff joints, infertility, PMS and Seasonal Affective Disorder (SAD). Excess sun threatens skin health, but insufficient light can disrupt the metabolism and hormonal balance, causing physical and psychological problems such as lethargy, depression and disturbed sleep patterns. Long hours in the office and lack of outdoor exercise may contribute to light deprivation, as artificial light fails to supply all the colours of the spectrum needed to maintain the body's physical and chemical equilibrium. Pure white light therapy restores the balance and also boosts vitamin D production. Twenty minutes to an hour of exposure to this white light has a positive, energising effect.

MAGNETO-THERAPY

Magnetotherapy is a 'battery-charging' system that uses electromagnetic fields to energise, speed up wound healing, and treat insomnia and lower back pain. (It is not suitable for those with pacemakers, pregnant women or cancer sufferers.) City life depletes the body's natural magnetism, resulting in slow circulation and lethargy. Research shows that blood circulation is stimulated by magnetic pads that attract electrically charged positive and negative ions in the bloodstream, which in turn improves the absorption of oxygen. Magnetotherapy involves relaxing on a magnetised couch for around 15 minutes. Patients may experience a slight tingling sensation, but nothing more.

NUTRITION THERAPY

Nutrition therapy encourages optimum health and corrects specific problems, including allergies, PMS, arthritis, asthma, eczema, chronic fatigue and migraine. Just as vitamin and mineral deficiencies lead to poor health, food intolerance also stresses the immune system and can cause full-blown allergy and illness. Nutritionists take a full inventory of your lifestyle, health status and eating habits. Then they test for food intolerances either by taking a blood sample, or by using a specialised machine. Adjusting your diet often means boosting your intake of specific nutrients or giving up certain foods. Avoiding certain foods gives your immune system a chance to recover and tackle other problems.

OSTEOPATHY TREATMENT

Osteopathy treats back and joint pain, aches and strains, sciatica, rheumatism, arthritis, injuries, PMS and asthma. It not only deals with bones, but the tendons, ligaments and muscles that hold them in place and enable them to move. Poor posture and repetitive strain throws this system out of balance, causing injury, restricted mobility and pain. Osteopathy aims to correct the balance by easing everything back into place. Most osteopaths adopt a gentle manipulative approach, beginning each session by checking your posture and areas of muscular tension. Then they position and support the body through a series of rhythmic movements and deep stretches to improve strength, posture and mobility.

POLARITY THERAPY

Polarity therapy balances health and energy to treat migraine, digestive problems, allergies, back pain and sciatica. Based on the theory that the body is like a living magnet, with energy currents flowing back and forth between positive and negative poles, it is a total balancing system that uses body work, nutrition, exercise and counselling. Part of the initial counselling involves recording everything you eat and drink for a week to help the therapist gauge your energy balance. Body work is like a combination of osteopathy, reflexology and Indian massage, with firm acupressure and joint manipulation. Dietary suggestions include plenty of fresh fruit and vegetable juices, and detoxing regimes are recommended.

QI GONG (CHI KUNG)

This technique treats stress, boosts energy and maintains mobility and balance. It is an ancient Chinese holistic exercise and meditation system that combines precise movements and breathing techniques. These cleanse the meridians (energy pathways) so that the vital life force, or *chi,* can flow freely. The almost balletic sequence of move- ments look effortless, but they are hard work at first. Qi gong is a discipline that re-educates you about the way you move and breathe. If you persevere, the experts say that you'll benefit from increased energy, mobility and poise. You won't lose weight, but your body shape may even change for the better. You will feel calmer and more stress-free.

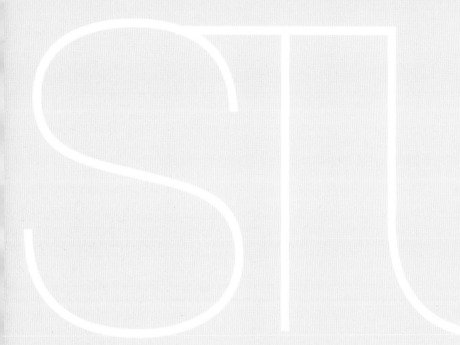

REFLEXOLOGY TREATMENT

Reflexology treats digestive problems, constipation, fluid retention, menstrual irregularities, PMS, menopausal symptoms, stress, fatigue, migraine and skin problems. It also maintains health and energy levels. The entire body is treated by massaging the reflex points in the feet and occasionally the hands. The body's six major meridians (energy pathways) all end in the feet, so each part of the foot relates to various body zones. The therapist applies firm finger and thumb pressure over the sole and around the heel and ankles to disperse congestion. You might feel a tingling or slightly sore sensation in the treated area. Most people experience the full benefits of reflexology the day after treatment.

SHIATSU TREATMENT

Shiatsu is a Japanese form of acupressure, or acupuncture without needles, which treats emotional and physical stress, back and shoulder tension, rheumatism, arthritis, digestive problems, migraine, asthma and insomnia. Points along the body's meridians (energy pathways) are stimulated to clear blockages and rebalance vital energy flow. Therapists say that this also disperses lactic acid and carbon monoxide that accumulate in muscles, alleviating stiffness and poor circulation. Freeing muscular tension also liberates the skeletal system and internal organs and often prompts emotional release. The massage can be quite vigorous, occasionally painful or extremely gentle.

TRADITIONAL CHINESE MEDICINE

Traditional Chinese medicine (TCM) treats skin problems, digestive disorders, menstrual and menopausal problems and chronic fatigue syndrome. TCM is an ancient tradition encompassing a complete health system, including diet, exercise (such as Tai Chi), acupuncture, and herbal remedies to maintain energy balance and facilitate the circulation of the life force, or *chi*. Yin and Yang, the fundamental principles of Chinese philosophy, are divided into eight principal patterns, such as hot and cold, and empty and full. These indicate bodily imbalances underlying disease. Therapists diagnose the imbalance and prescribe the appropriate treatment to re-establish the optimum energy flow and the Yin/Yang balance.

USUI METHOD REIKI

Reiki is beneficial for relaxation, muscular strain, general aches and immune-related conditions such as HIV. A hands-on healing system developed in the mid-1800s by a Japanese doctor of philosophy, Mikao Usui, reiki loosely means the free flow of universal energy, or *ki*. It is an eclectic system that owes much to Buddhist thought. Practitioners believe they act as conductors, transferring universal energy to the patient via their hands. This energy then has a balancing effect on both body and mind. The practitioner rests his/her hands on key points over the entire head and body of the patient. Treatments can have a deeply calming, relaxing or energising effect, depending on the patient's needs.

VOICE THERAPY

Voice therapy helps to dispel stress and encourage self-expression through non-verbal communication. It has proved especially useful in treating autism and learning difficulties. During therapy, sounds are made that are an invaluable means of communication (they can have a far more powerful effect than intellectually charged words). Working on the basis that you don't have to be a singer with perfect pitch to use your voice as a satisfying medium for emotional release, the noises include chanting, singing or simply 'mouth music' – sounds made instinctively to describe or dispel emotion. The sounds resonate through the entire body and have an inspiring, energising and relaxing effect.

WATER THERAPY

Water therapy eases muscular tension, joint pain, rheumatism, arthritis, bronchitis and chronic fatigue syndrome. (Avoid this type of treatment if you have heart disease or high blood pressure.) Also known as hydrotherapy, 'taking the waters' is an important part of naturopathic medicine dating at least to ancient Greek, Roman and Celtic times. The curative, immune-boosting effect of hot and cold mineral spring baths forms the basis of spa treatments all over the world. The many forms of treatment exploit water in all its forms and include steam rooms and Turkish baths, balneotherapy (total immersion in varying degrees of warm and cold water), contrast bathing, foot baths and thalassotherapy.

YOGA TECHNIQUES

Yoga is ideal for relaxation, mind and body tuning, and postural and muscular control. *Asanas*, or postures, are gentle stretches that promote balance, strength, control and flexibility. They work out the entire body, including internal organs, which are massaged by specific movements. Breathing is also integral to yoga. According to the Indian sage Paanjali, who lived over 2000 years ago, there are eight yogic steps to enlightenment. These include moral responsibility, self-discipline and meditation as well as the familiar postures. The many Western yoga techniques concentrate on body conditioning. Power and dynamis yoga, for example, combine aerobic techniques with traditional stretching.

ZERO BALANCING

This technique treats neck and back pain, stress, migraines and sports injuries. It is a combination of hands-on healing and energy balancing that aims to soothe, stretch and balance both physical and mental energies, and to provide mind, body and soul healing. Theoretically, the body has three energy fields: an aura-like background energy; a worldly vertical energy that gives a sense of space; and an internal energy circulation. Physical and emotional trauma can affect these energy circulations and zero balancing clears blockages and eases the flow. Manipulation is bone-deep and involves the entire body. Often this physical manipulation releases emotional memory, which may be the underlying cause of stress.

VITAMINS AND MINERALS

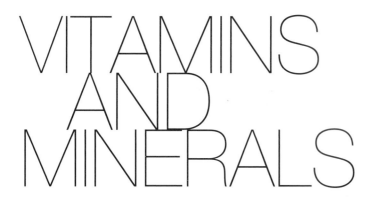

Even if your diet is well-balanced and nutritious, the effects of modern living can deplete essential vitamin and mineral reserves. Find the best natural sources of vitamins and minerals and ensure your recommended daily intake (RDI) is correct.

VITAMIN A

Essential for good vision, healthy skin, growth and resistance to infection. It can also be beneficial for acne sufferers. Sources: liver, oily fish, dairy produce and egg yolk. Some beta-carotene (from green fruit, oranges and vegetables such as carrots and spinach) is converted into vitamin A by the body. RDI: 750mcg, equivalent to one carrot. Exceeding this can cause dry, itchy skin, loss of appetite and nausea.

VITAMIN B1 (THIAMINE)

Vital for energy production and the metabolism of sugar. Deficiencies can cause depression, anxiety, poor appetite, nausea and personality changes. Women on the pill, breast-feeding mothers and those who consume too much sugar and alcohol could be deficient. Sources: meat, fish, nuts, wholegrains, sesame seeds. RDI: 0.8–1.1mg

VITAMIN B12 (CYANOCOBALAMIN)

Required for the formation of red blood cells, nerve cells and genetic material (DNA). Vitamin B12 also maintains the functioning of the nervous system. Vegans and those who suffer from anaemia can be deficient. Sources: meat, liver, eggs, milk and yeast extract. RDI: 2mcg

VITAMIN C (ASCORBIC ACID)

Required for healthy bones, teeth and gums, the formation of collagen, and healing and repair of tissues. Vitamin C is also essential for the absorption of iron within the body. Smoking cigarettes depletes vitamin C supplies. Deficiencies can be detected in skin that bruises easily. Sources: citrus fruits, capsicum, broccoli, spinach and cabbage. RDI: 30–40mg. Excess vitamin C can cause diarrhoea and increase the risk of kidney stones.

VITAMIN D

Necessary for muscle strength and the balance of calcium in bones and teeth. Malnutrition and lack of daylight can contribute to deficiencies. Sources: milk, margarine, sardines, cod liver oil, eggs and sunlight. RDI: not specified in Australia due to the available sunlight.

VITAMIN E

Protects tissues from general wear and tear and helps to prevent fats and cholesterol from causing damage to the organs. Sources: seafood, most nuts, seeds and vegetables. RDI: 7–10mg

FOLIC ACID

Helps to maintain the nervous system, essential for healthy blood and especially important for child-bearing women. Sources: all green leafy vegetables, liver, kidney, avocado, watercress, bran and fortified cereals. RDI: 200mcg

VITAMIN B2 (RIBOFLAVIN)

Essential for energy production and for healthy skin and eyes. Deficiencies can be detected by mild fatigue and a red ring around the iris. Sources: milk, cheese, yoghurt, almonds, green vegetables, mushrooms. RDI: 1.2–1.7mg

VITAMIN B3 (NIACIN)

Necessary for the metabolism of carbohydrates and used medically to lower cholesterol levels. Sources: meat, fish, liver, tuna, peanuts. RDI: 13–19mg

VITAMIN B6 (PYRIDOXINE)

Needed for the formation of red blood cells and metabolism of protein. Often used to treat PMS, morning sickness and hormonal imbalances. Smoking and eating junk food increases the probability of B6 deficiencies. Sources: meat, poultry, fish, bananas, avocado, soybeans, nuts, wholegrains, vegetables. RDI: 0.9mg–1.9mg

CALCIUM

Necessary for strong bones and teeth and to maintain the functioning of the nerves and muscles. Lack of calcium is linked to osteoporosis (bone thinning). Exercising reduces the body's rate of calcium loss. If you are going through menopause or don't eat dairy produce, you could be deficient in calcium. Sources: milk, cheese, sardines, beans, green vegetables. RDI: 800mg

ZINC

Essential for normal growth, healthy skin, mental health and hormone production. Eczema, acne, greasy or dry facial skin are symptoms linked to zinc deficiencies. Coffee and tea drinkers, vegetarians and long-term users of diuretics are susceptible to low levels of zinc. Sources: meat, wholegrains, nuts, pumpkin seeds, eggs, carrots, ginger, beans and lentils. RDI: 12mg

IRON

Required to manufacture haemoglobin (the pigment in red blood cells that carries oxygen to all parts of the body), and for energy production. Lack of iron causes fatigue, low energy levels, depression, poor digestion and can be detected by brittle nails, a pale complexion, heavy periods and recurrent thrush. Sources: meat, liver, oysters, wholegrains, nuts, eggs and fortified breakfast cereals. RDI: 15–16mg

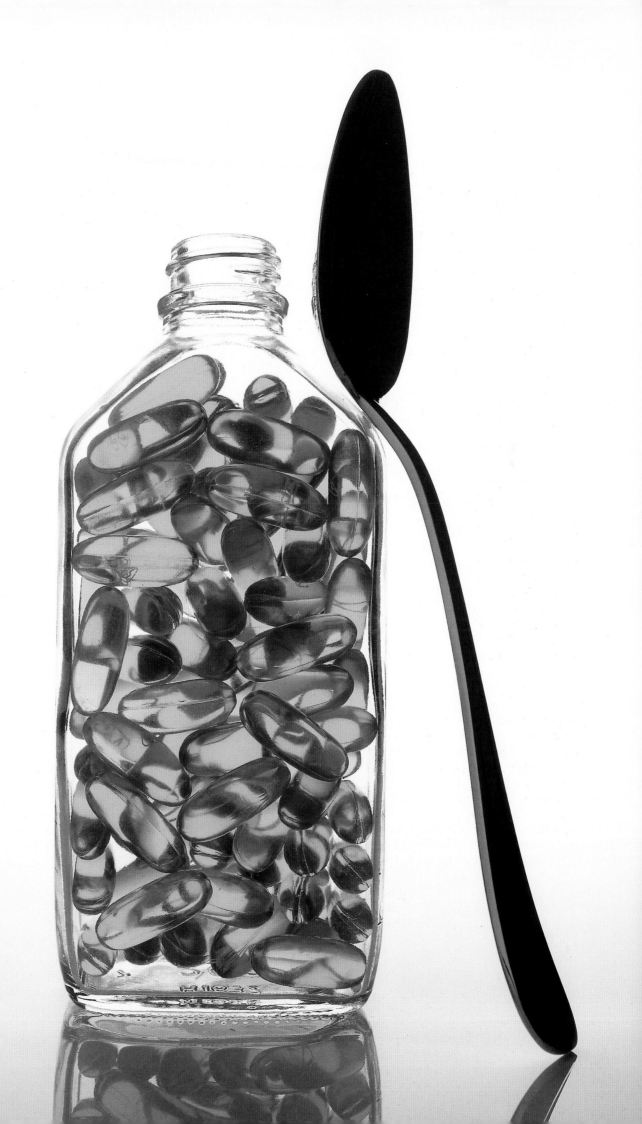

IMPROVE INNER HEALTH

FOLLOW THESE STEPS TO IMPROVE YOUR WELL-BEING

BANISH PMS

If you suffer from PMS, eliminate dairy produce from your diet for seven days before your period. Also increase your intake of magnesium, vitamin B6, B complex and beta-carotene. Cut down your intake of salt and caffeine and steer clear of alcohol.

STRONG BACK

Prevent back pain by improving your work station. Ensure your desk is the correct height and your chair offers the best support. When bending down, always bend from the knees (don't stoop over). If you have back pain, see an osteopath.

EASE PAIN

When a headache kicks in, try soaking your feet in a bowl of warm water mixed with a teaspoon of cayenne pepper for 10 minutes. This will draw the blood away from your head down to your feet, relax your body and ease the pain of a headache.

VITAMIN THERAPY

Increase your intake of bioflavonoids (the chemicals found in lemons, plums, grape-fruits and blackberries) and vitamin C to reduce the appearance of broken capillaries on the skin. These substances strengthen the walls of the capillaries.

MORNING AFTER

Alcohol depletes the body's vital supply of vitamins B and C. The best hangover cures contain citrus juices which are rich in natural sugars and vitamin C, celery and apple juice to help rebalance the body, and beetroot to cleanse the kidneys.

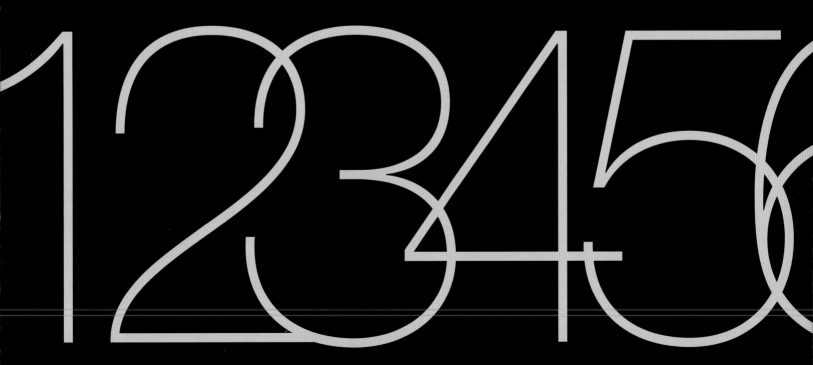

ADULT ACNE

A sudden outbreak of adult acne can occur due to hormonal imbalances, often triggered by stress. To treat the condition. consult an endocrin-ologist or your doctor for an androgen blood test so that medication can be prescribed.

YEAST PROBLEM

If you suffer from recurrent candida (thrush), avoid wearing tight clothing and nylon underwear, shower rather than bath, use unperfumed toiletries, and non-biological washing powder, reduce sugar consumption and opt for a yeast-free diet.

HAY FEVER

If you suffer from hay fever, look at ways of avoiding exposure to potential allergens such as pets and flowers. Increase your intake of kiwi fruit, blackcurrants and citrus fruits to help relieve congestion. They will also have a natural anti-inflammatory effect.

HEALTH ISSUE

Endometriosis, which is linked with long, heavy periods and painful intercourse, affects one in 10 women. Involving the erratic growth of the cells lining the uterus, it can be treated with the pill, anti-inflammatory analgesics or laparo-scopic therapy.

PERFECT TIMING

If you're having an operation, you should ideally have it on or around the time you ovulate. Studies have revealed that women who have operations between days 13 and 21 of their menstrual cycle make a much speedier recovery.

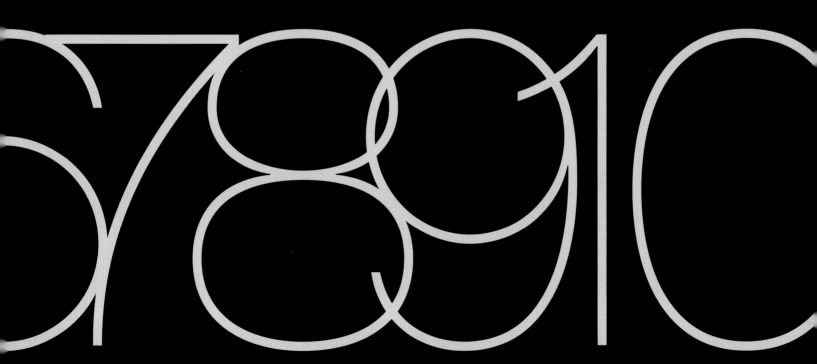

PROBLEM

What is the most effective way to boost your iron intake?

Have a fresh juice incorporating spinach or green, leafy vegetables. This is more beneficial to the body than taking iron tablets.

Do you feel bloated after meals?

To aid digestion, try drinking a cup of peppermint tea after you eat.

Can a low-fat diet **benefit your looks?**

A low-fat diet will keep you in trim and help prevent age spots from developing later in life.

How can you sustain good health?

The experts recommend exposing yourself to at least two hours of natural light a day to maintain optimum health. Incorporate this factor into your exercise regime.

Is it possible to overdose on vitamins?

Always stick to the recommended dose. Excessive intake of some vitamins can be dangerous.

Are your nails prone to breakages?

Make sure you are obtaining enough calcium, iron and zinc from your diet to maintain healthy, strong nails. Good foods to eat include raw vegetables, fresh fruits and dairy produce.

Is there a way to ensure the longevity of vitamin pills?

After you open a bottle of vitamin pills, throw away the ball of cotton wool that comes inside the bottle. It can attract moisture and damage or contaminate the pills.

Do you feel nauseous when travelling?

To ease motion sickness, try eating foods containing ginger.

Is there a quick-fix remedy for an upset stomach?

Drinking a mixture of bicarbonate of soda and water will help to settle your stomach.

How can you treat dry and brittle hair?

Strengthen your hair by increasing your intake of iron and vitamins A and B.

SOLUTION

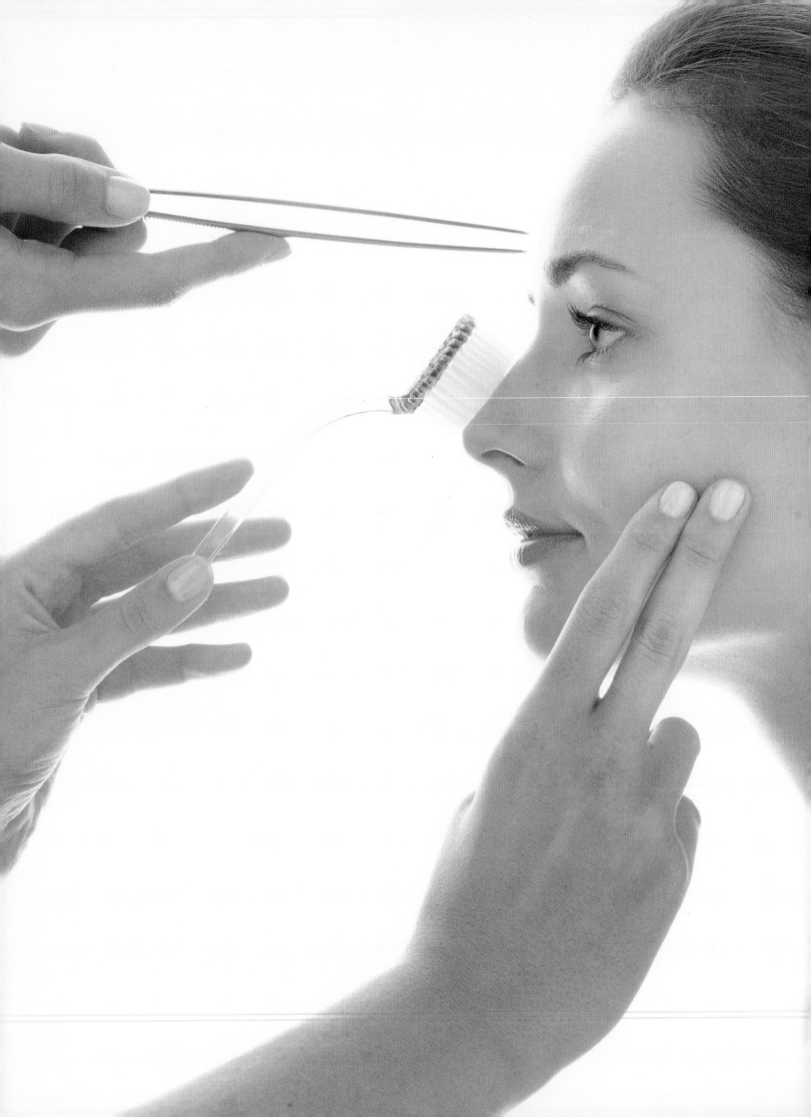

SKIN 2

SKIN SHOULD BE A PRIZED ASSET. A HEALTHY DIET, SUFFICIENT SLEEP, REGULAR EXERCISE AND A COMPREHENSIVE BEAUTY REGIME ARE ALL ESSENTIAL TO MAINTAIN FLAWLESS SKIN.

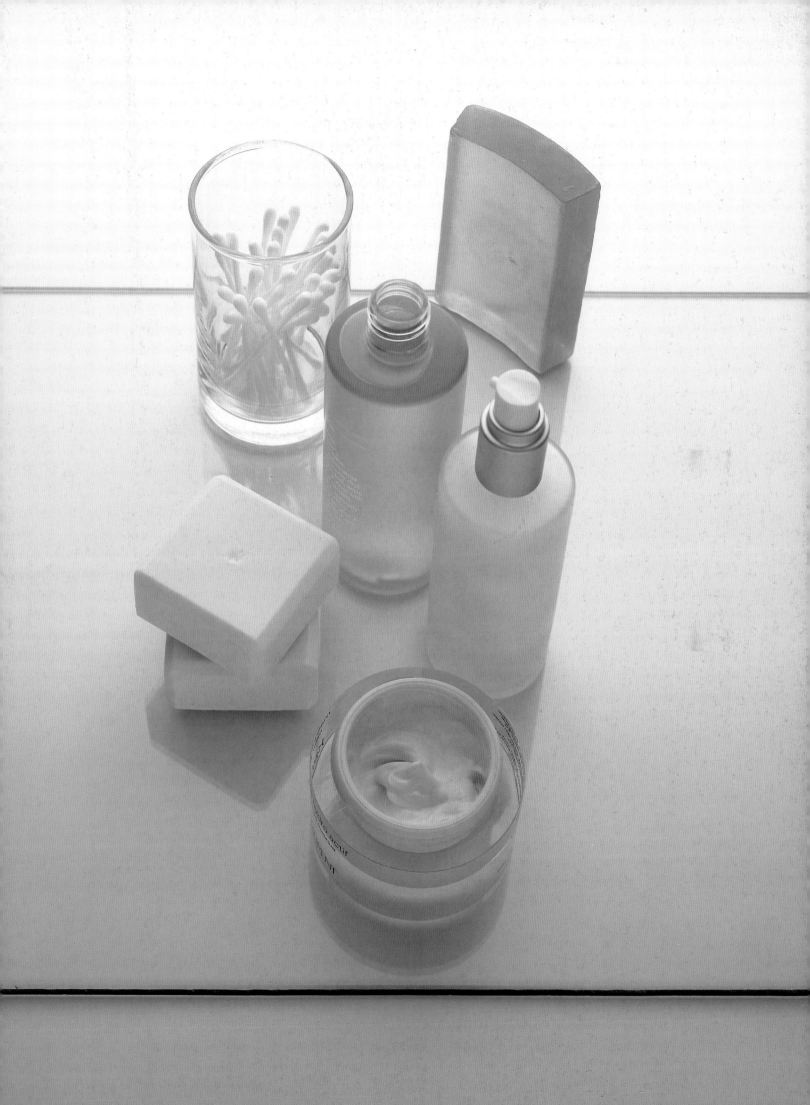

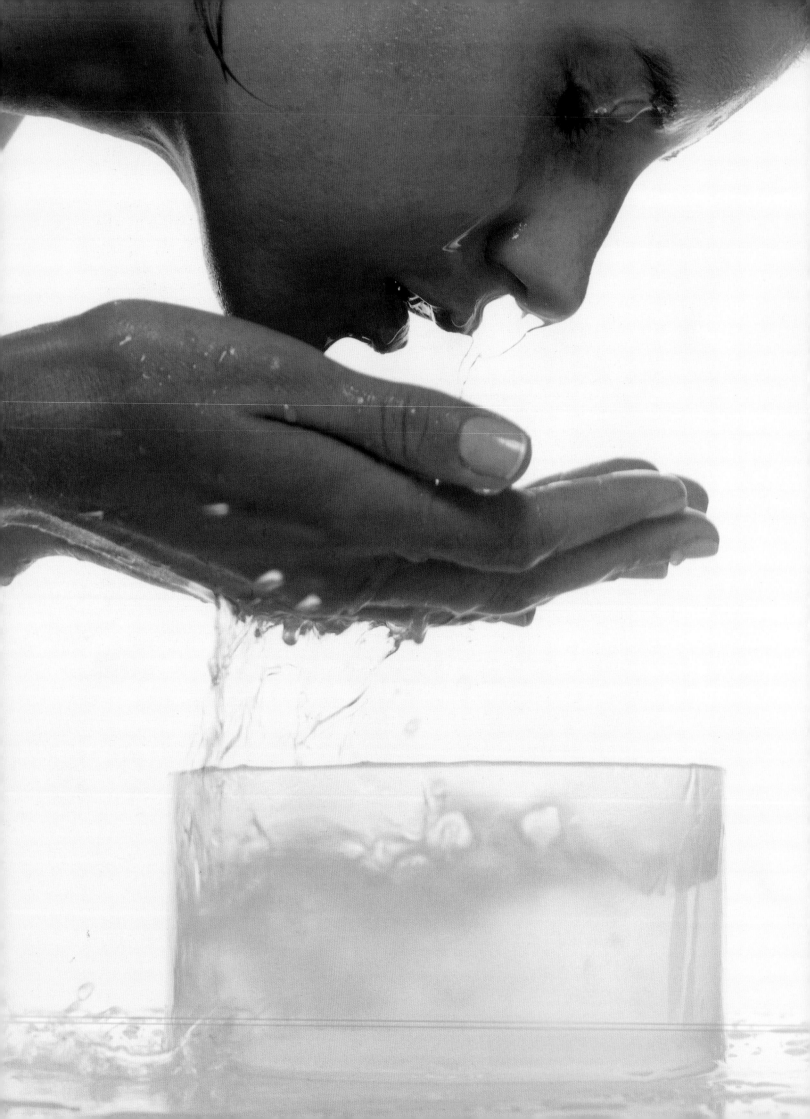

SKINCARE

The skin's needs change from season to season, and with age, hormonal fluctuations, diet and lifestyle. Finding products to suit these requirements can often be a costly, hit-and-miss affair. To make skincare simple, first identify your skin type and then address its needs.

NORMAL SKIN has an even tone, a smooth texture, no visible pores or blemishes, and no greasy patches or flaky areas. A basic beauty regime is sufficient to maintain its natural balance, but don't be tempted to neglect your skin, a great-looking complexion won't last forever.

SENSITIVE SKIN is commonly dry, delicate and prone to allergic reactions. Temperature changes, some detergents, cosmetics and alcohol (used on the skin) can all cause irritation, leaving the skin red and blotchy, with visible surface veins. Choose products that do not contain potential allergens such as fragrance or PABA sunscreens.

OILY SKIN is characterised by an over-production of sebum (the skin's natural hydrator), which results in spots and blemishes. The great advantage of this skin type is that it ages at a slower rate than other skin types. Avoid harsh products that strip your skin of oil and encourage flakiness. They can cause a reaction known as reactive seborrhoea, where the oil glands work overtime to compensate for the loss of natural oils. Products that leave your skin feeling taut and dehydrated should also be avoided, as they cause the upper layers of the skin to shrink. This restricts oil flow through the pores and leads to blockages and breakouts. To cleanse oily skin, use oil-based products as they dissolve sebum effectively. Opt for oil-free moisturisers to maintain a shine-free complexion.

DRY SKIN has a low level of sebum and can be prone to sensitivity. Dryness is exacerbated by wind, extremes of temperature and airconditioning, all of which cause the skin to flake, chap and feel tight. Use moisture-rich products and increase the intake of essential fatty acids in your diet. If you have dry skin, use a cream- or oil-based cleanser. Avoid water-soluble variants as exposing dry skin to water can aggravate the condition.

SKIN SOLUTIONS

A healthy diet is essential for healthy skin. Vitamin C is required for collagen production; beta-carotene is converted into vitamin A, a substance essential for maintaining skin tissue; vitamin E is vital for skin condition; and vitamin B helps repair the skin.

Evening primrose oil

supplements are beneficial for skin. They contain gamma-linolenic acid (GLA), an essential fatty acid reputed to strengthen skin cells and boost their moisture content.

Get sufficient sleep as the skin's

cellular repair activity is at its optimum during this resting phase.

Exercise benefits skin as it boosts

circulation and encourages blood flow. Regular exercise will nourish and cleanse your skin from within.

SKIN SOLUTIONS

To cleanse the eye area, don't use your normal cleanser. Look for special oil-free eye make-up removers. They contain scientifically tested ingredients that won't irritate the delicate eye area.

After cleansing, gently splash your face with cold water. This is a great pick-me-up in the mornings and will jump-start the skin's circulation.

Avoid exfoliating the skin on your face if you have networks of surface veins, it can intensify the problem.

For a skin-reviving treat, decant some toner into a plastic spray bottle and store it in the fridge. Use it when required as a skin booster or as a cooling treat in summer.

CLEANSING

When you choose a cleanser, consider your skin type and your personal preferences. Also bear in mind that cleanser is only ever on the skin for little more than 30 seconds. An effective cleanser should remove impurities without leaving any residue or greasy film on your skin once it is removed.

AVOID CLEANSING WITH SOAP AND WATER. Skin is slightly acidic whereas soap is alkaline – it disrupts the skin's naturally acidic protective film. An oil-based cleanser is suitable for all skin types and removes make-up effectively. Water-soluble and oil-based cleansers are ideal for oily and combination skins. Cream cleansers suit dry skins. If you have sensitive skin, avoid cleansers rich in fragrance, colour and any potential skin irritants.

WHEN APPLYING AN OIL-BASED OR CREAM CLEANSER, smooth it on, leave it for a few seconds to dissolve impurities and then gently wipe it off with a damp tissue or cotton wool. If you're using wash-off cleanser, apply it to damp skin and then rinse with warm water. Removing cleanser with a facial sponge or cleansing brush will remove impurities and exfoliate the skin at the same time.

EXFOLIATING

Skin constantly produces new cells and sheds old ones. Normal skin renews its cells every 28 days. This process slows down with age, and leaves the complexion looking dull and lifeless. Exfoliating scrubs, creams or gels whisk away dead skin cells and the manual pressure exerted during exfoliation peps up circulation and helps stimulate cell production. Exfoliate your face every two to three days. If you have acne or sensitive skin, use a peel-off face mask instead of an exfoliator.

TONING

Using toner after cleansing is optional. It will refresh your skin and remove any impurities or remnants of cleanser. Avoid alcohol-based toner even if you have an oily complexion, as it strips the skin of essential moisture. Floral waters are inexpensive alternatives to commercial toners: witch-hazel is ideal for oily, problem skin; rose water for dry complexions; and camomile water suits both normal and sensitive skins.

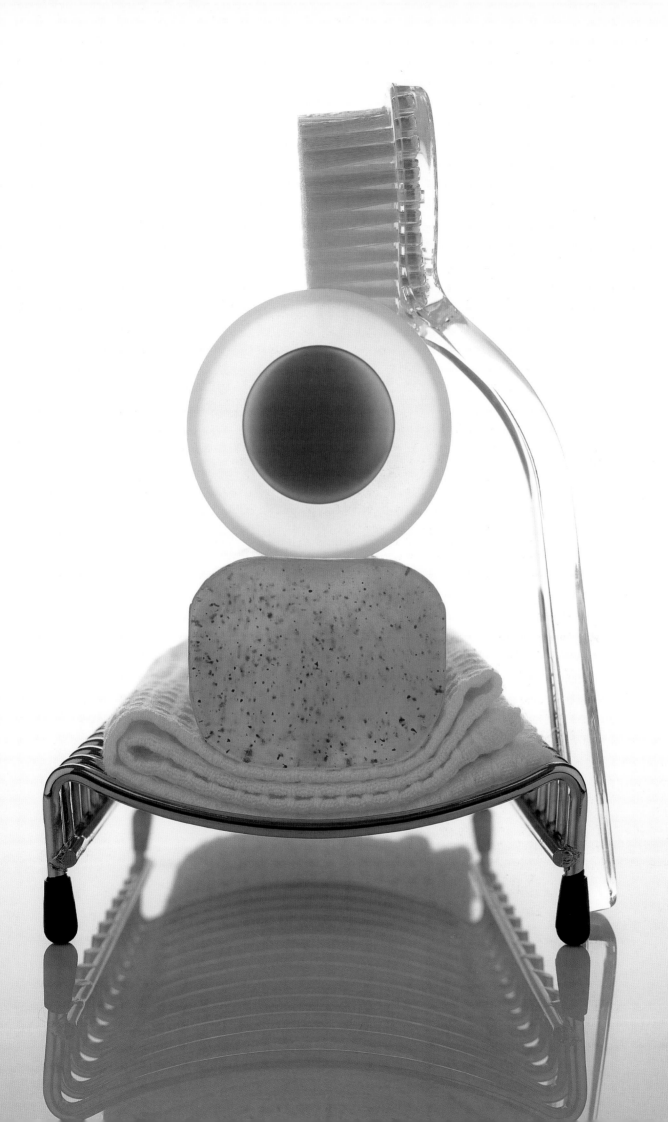

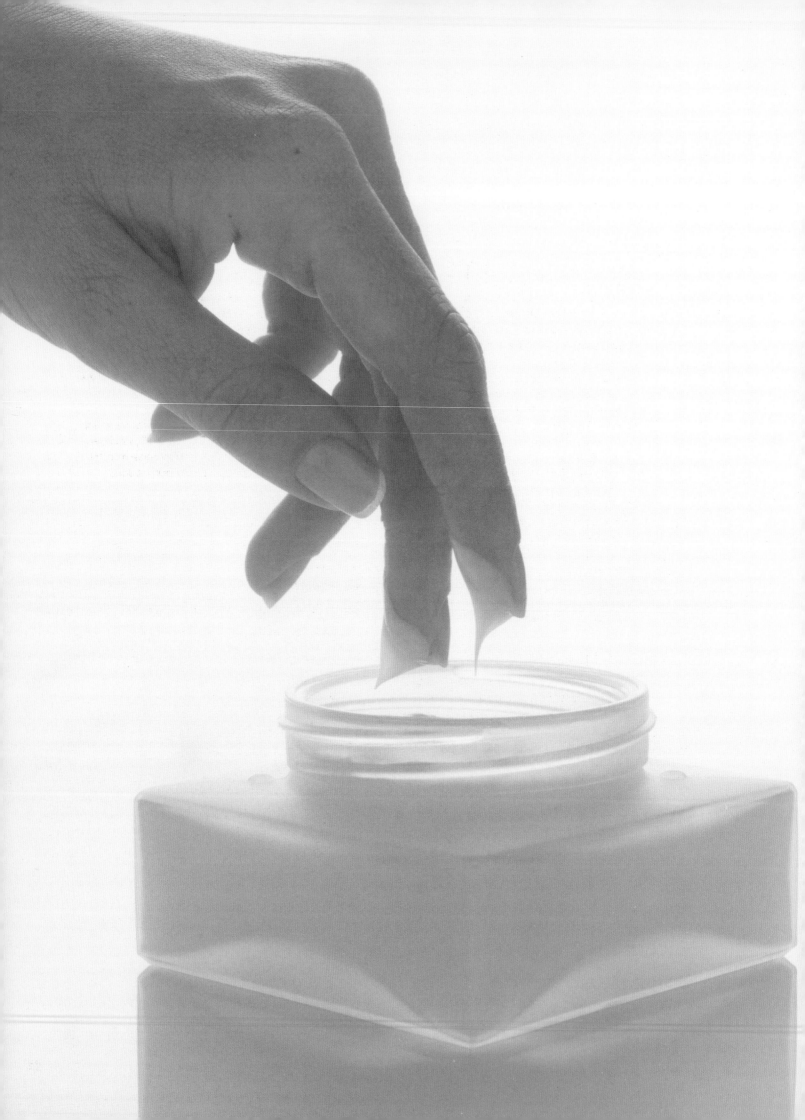

SKIN SOLUTIONS

To apply moisturiser, pat it onto your skin instead of smoothing it on. This increases circulation and invigorates your complexion.

During the day use a moisturiser containing sunscreen and smooth on a preparation enriched with antioxidants or alpha hydroxy acids at night.

While steaming your face, protect the delicate skin around your eyes with a film of moisturiser.

To zap pimples and blemishes, dab tea-tree or lavender oil (which both have anti-bacterial properties) onto the affected area with a cotton bud.

MOISTURISING

Your skin has a natural moisturising factor (NMF) that regulates water flow from the dermis (the skin's deepest layer) to the surface. Sebum (the skin's natural hydrator) also plays a vital role in the prevention of moisture loss, forming a barrier on the surface of the skin that delays water evaporation. With age, both the NMF and sebum production decrease, hence the need for a water-regulating moisturiser. All skin types, even those prone to oiliness, need moisturising twice a day.

THERE ARE TWO TYPES OF MOISTURISERS: humectants and occlusives. Humectants draw water up from the depths of the dermis or attract it from the surrounding atmosphere. Occlusives create an oily film on the skin's surface to seal in moisture and prevent it from evaporating into the atmosphere.

CHOOSE A MOISTURISER TO SUIT YOUR SKIN TYPE: oil-free formulas and oil-in-water emulsions benefit oily skins, and water-in-oil formulations, which are more hydrating, suit dry/normal skins. Always spritz your skin with water before applying moisturiser. The water 'plumps' up the skin cells, creating an even surface and makes lines less apparent, and the moisturiser prevents this water from evaporating. Today's advanced formulations can maintain this effect for up to 12 hours.

STEAMING

Giving your face a steam or sauna is a good deep-cleansing treat, especially for congested skin. Remove all make-up and cleanse your skin. Fill a bowl with near-boiling water and add three drops of each essential oil recommended for your skin type: for normal skin use lavender and mandarin; for dry skin use camomile and rose; for oily skin lemon and eucalyptus; and for combination skin lavender and cypress. Once you've added the oils, agitate the water to disperse the droplets. Hold your face about 20–30cm above the bowl and place a towel over your head and the bowl for three minutes. This opens the pores and prepares your skin for the application of a face mask.

AVOID THIS TREATMENT IF YOU HAVE SENSITIVE SKIN or broken capillaries on your face. The intense heat of the water causes the blood vessels under the surface of the skin to dilate, exacerbating the problem. Facial steaming is not recommended if you are pregnant or suffer from asthma.

FACE MASKS

Use a face mask once a week. For the best results, apply the mask after a facial steam and leave it on only for the time specified by the manufacturer.

WHEN CHOOSING A MASK, bear the following in mind: mud- or clay-enriched masks are ideal for deep-cleansing the skin. They contain negatively charged ions, which attract positively charged impurities. Gel-based masks set to form a fine film, which when washed away removes dead cells and grime. Rich cream masks (which do not set) are beneficial for dry and mature skins. Sulphur-based masks treat oily and problem skins but should not be used on sensitive or dry skins. Fast-acting masks are an option when you're pushed for time.

EYE CARE

Because the skin around your eyes is much thinner than the skin on the rest of your face, it requires extra care, especially to ward off signs of ageing. Use an eye cream or gel both at night and in the morning. Only apply it along the orbital bone (the bone directly under the eye). Gently pat it on, being careful not to drag the skin.

DARK CIRCLES UNDER YOUR EYES can be the result of poor circulation, medication, illness or toxin build-up; they can also be hereditary. The skin in this area is thin, so the blood vessels lie close to the surface, giving it a blue-black tint. If the blood vessels leak, darker, even permanent, discolouration can occur. Dark circles can be camouflaged with concealer, or permanently lightened by a chemical peel, an extremely painful process.

PUFFINESS AROUND YOUR EYES is caused by a build-up of toxins or excess fluids. To help reduce any swelling, stimulate your lymphatic system by pressing gently along the eyebrow and around the eye socket with your middle finger. For a cooling and soothing effect, store an eye cream or gel in the fridge and gently pat it onto the delicate skin around your eyes.

LIP CARE

Lips lack several of the body's protective substances, so they need extra protection. Without an effective lipid barrier, they lose moisture regularly; their lack of hydrating sebaceous glands makes them prone to chapping and dryness; and, lacking melanin (the body's natural protector), they burn easily.

WEAR PROTECTIVE LIP BALM enriched with a sun filter or lipstick with a high SPF when outdoors. To maintain the condition of your lips, coat them with Vaseline and then gently exfoliate using a clean toothbrush.

SKIN SOLUTIONS

Treat your eyes while you have a face mask on. Soak two cotton-wool pads in cold camomile tea and place them over your eyes.

Treat sore eyes caused by exposure to the sun, wind or chlorine with a soothing eye bath. Try blending 1–2 tablespoons of rose water with 150ml distilled water to bathe your eyes.

Avoid taking antibiotics if possible as they destroy intestinal bacteria, which are essential for healthy skin. If you take antibiotics, counterbalance their effects by eating foods rich in vitamin B.

Keep your lips hydrated with lip balm and make sure the surrounding skin is sufficiently moisturised to prevent lines from appearing around your mouth.

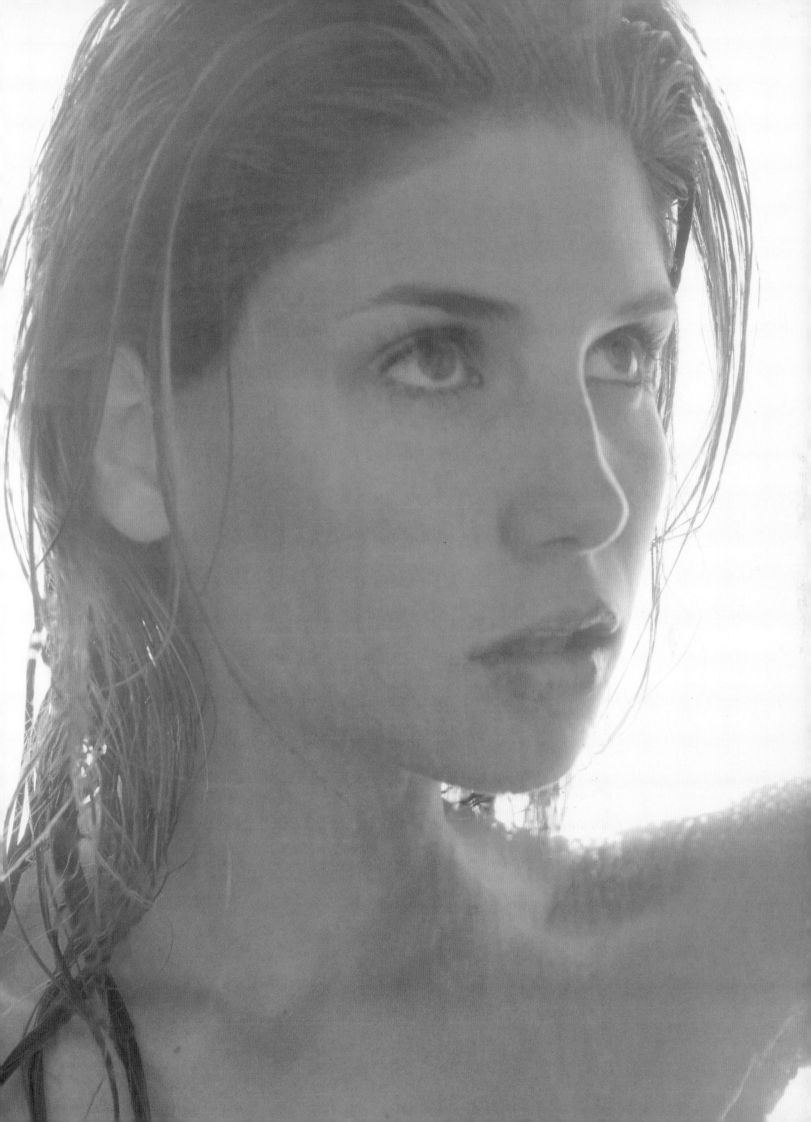

CHANGING FACES

ADDRESS YOUR SKIN'S NEEDS AS YOU AGE

20s 30s

IN YOUR 20s, since cell turnover is at its best, your complexion should be in optimum condition after undergoing major changes in the teenage years. If your skin is functioning properly, a basic skincare regime is sufficient. Avoid soaps as they have a dehydrating effect, so look for pH-balanced cleansing bars instead. Toner is optional and use a moisturiser regularly. Pay close attention to your neck, throat and hands when applying moisturiser and look after the delicate skin around your eyes.

IF YOU SUNBATHED REGULARLY as a teenager, damage to your skin's blueprint cells may already have been done. Take preventative measures by wearing sunscreen daily.

SKIN PRONE TO EXCESSIVE OILINESS and pimples is often a result of hormones that are still stabilising. Opt for oil-free skincare products and cosmetics. Steaming your face regularly and applying face masks will also benefit congested skin.

IN YOUR 30s, cell turnover and sebum production decrease and lines and wrinkles become more obvious. Exfoliate your skin at least twice a week and use a hydrating mask once a week. Use an eye-care preparation at night and in the morning.

PIGMENTATION PROBLEMS are common during these years as the skin becomes less efficient at manufacturing melanin. Brown patches known as melasma or chloasma can appear around the eyes, lips, cheeks and forehead during pregnancy, or as a result of hormonal changes, exposure to the sun or taking the contraceptive pill. There are various options to treat uneven skin tone. Creams containing hydroquinone, a substance that temporarily halts pigment production, help the condition. Retina A is also an option for treating hyper-pigmentation but if your skin is sensitive, it can actually cause further darkening. Laser resurfacing can also be used to remove patches of uneven skin tone.

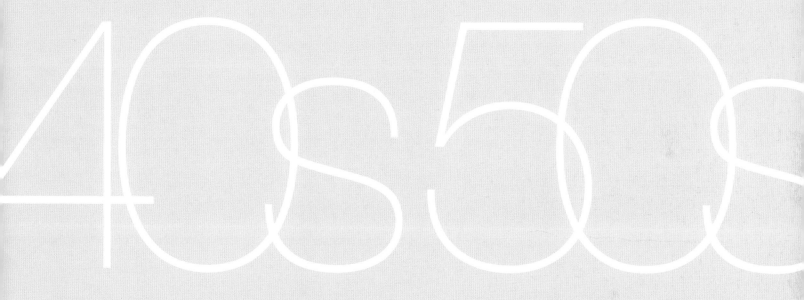

IN YOUR 40s, the protective film on the skin's surface becomes less effective at retaining moisture. This causes a much higher percentage of water loss, which leads to dryness. Apply moisturiser twice a day and look for preparations such as firming serums that offer the skin extra reinforcement.

FINE LINES, WRINKLES, BROKEN VEINS and dull skin can be made less apparent with chemical peels or regular facials. Exfoliate your skin and treat both your face and eyes to treatment masks twice a week. Use a cream cleanser instead of a water-soluble type, as constantly wetting and drying your face will only step up moisture loss. Increase your intake of antioxidants by eating fresh fruits and vegetables or by taking a daily vitamin supplement.

SUN OR AGE SPOTS on the face can treated with creams containing retinoic acid, hydroquinone, glycolic or kojic acid. They can also be eradicated by chemical peels and laser treatments.

IN YOUR 50s, cell turnover decreases by almost 50%, the production of sebum for natural hydration slows down and the skin's outer layer becomes less resilient. After the menopause, oestrogen (the skin's youth hormone) production slows down and the skin becomes much drier. Oestrogen diminishes collagen (the skin's structural support system), making the skin thinner. Using a product enriched with an alpha hydroxy acid is believed to boost the production of collagen. Look for moisture-rich products, use a cream cleanser, avoid alcohol-based toners and opt for specialist products to care for your eyes and lips. Ensure that you drink sufficient amounts of water each day.

AS THE SKIN'S RESILIENCE BREAKS DOWN, broken capillaries can appear on the surface. These can be treated with a course of laser resurfacing or sclerotherapy, in which a solution is injected into the vein, causing it to recede.

PREVENT SKIN AGEING

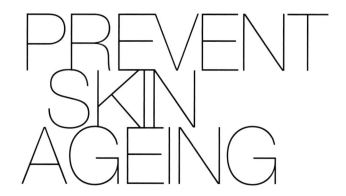

There are two types of skin ageing: intrinsic ageing, the natural, biological process which is beyond our control; and extrinsic ageing, which is caused by factors including environmental aggressors, diet, lifestyle, medication and stress. In the past, anti-ageing procedures were limited. Now there are relatively simple measures on offer which give results that are comparable to a surgical facelift.

MASSAGE

If you include simple massage movements in your existing beauty regime, you will see the benefits in a couple of months. When applying moisturiser, try lightly circling your hands up from your chin to the centre of your forehead and gliding each hand down each side of your face, repeating 12 times. To keep facial lines from setting in around your mouth, over-exaggerate smiling, and then gnash your teeth together. Repeat each motion 24 times. To prevent a wrinkled neck, sweep your hands up under your chin and down again. Repeat 12 times.

MUSCLE TONING

Electrotherapy involves the stimulation of the under-lying muscles of the face with a mild, painless electric current. This treatment is costly and requires constant maintenance sessions after the initial course.

PRESSURE POINTS

The acupuncture facelift is one of the more unusual alternatives to surgery. This treatment aims to rebalance the body's energy flow and also improve the appearance of the skin, tone the facial muscles and step up circulation. Normally 12 needles are inserted at specific regions of the face (just below the skin's surface), which address the body's inner health and outer beauty. It's a pain-free procedure that leaves you feeling as good as you look. For best results, a course of these facials is recommended.

ANTIOXIDANTS

Skin is constantly under attack from free radicals, rogue molecules that accelerate premature ageing. Vitamins E and C and beta-carotene are antioxidants that help put a stop to free radical activity. All working in slightly different ways, the overall effect of antioxidants is to mop up free radicals as they form, preventing them from doing serious damage within the body. Antioxidants in creams will protect the skin from environmental factors, while antioxidants taken orally, in tablet form or from foods such as fresh fruits and vegetables help to neutralise the by-products of this oxidation process. Antioxidants should be an integral part of any anti-ageing regime.

LYMPH STIMULATION

Women can suffer from water retention on both the face and body. Stimulating the lymphatic system helps address this problem. Lymphatic drainage facials help reshape the face by reducing puffiness around the eyes, cheeks and chin.

LINE FILLERS

For those who want to lessen the appearance of wrinkles caused by frowning and scowling, line-filling injections are an option. Synthetic collagen or the body's own fat, which is removed from an area such as the hips or thighs, is injected into wrinkles. The results are short-term, as collagen is absorbed into the body within three months and only some of the fat remains permanent. To maintain effects, top-up treatments are essential.

AHAs

Alpha hydroxy acids (AHAs) or fruit acids are naturally occurring compounds that break down the inter-cellular cement causing redundant skin cells to stick together. With regular use, AHAs improve overall skin texture and make ageing skins look more radiant. They are also reputed to boost the production of collagen and hyaluronic acid (the skin's natural water-retaining substance). For the best results, users of AHAs should avoid washing their skins with alkaline soaps. Preparations enriched with AHAs should be applied to cleansed skin and left for 10 minutes before further preparations are applied to the face.

CHEMICAL PEELS

High concentrates of alpha hydroxy acids are used to peel off the outer layers of the skin, removing fine lines and wrinkles. The concentration of acids used ranges from 15% strength, commonly used in beauty salons, to 70% strength, administered by surgeons and dermatologists for severely damaged and mature skins. Recovery periods vary depending on the strength of the peel. It can be a painful process but it does result in younger, smoother skin.

LASER RESURFACING

A good alternative to surgery, laser resurfacing removes the outer layers of old, wrinkled or sun-damaged skin. It can also treat age spots and uneven skin tone. This non-invasive treatment is more accurate and less painful than the surgeon's knife, and the skin heals faster than if you've had cosmetic surgery. Recovery periods vary, usually 10 days after a treatment the skin is red but can be concealed with make-up. Within six weeks it will have healed totally.

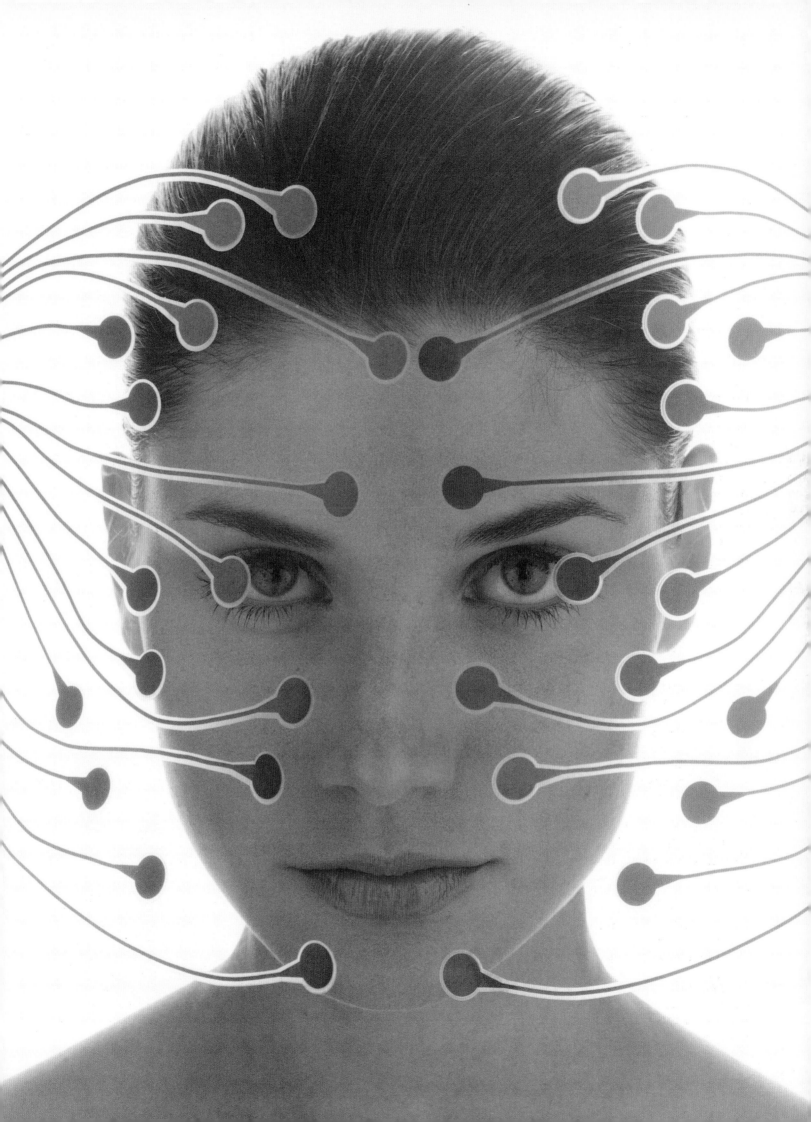

HEALTHY SKIN

FOLLOW THESE STEPS TO ACHIEVE A RADIANT COMPLEXION

DETOX DRINK

Start your day with a cup of boiling water laced with the juice of half a lemon. This drink flushes out any impurities that may have built up in your system overnight. Lemon also acts as a gentle cleanser for the liver.

FADDISH FOODS

Apart from piling on the pounds, certain fats actually accelerate ageing because they increase free radical activity within the body. Avoid polyunsaturated fats, which are found mainly in processed foods and in peanut, safflower and corn oils.

KEEP SMILING

On average, children smile 400 times a day, while adults only manage 15. Smiling tightens the supporting connective tissue around your mouth which helps to maintain the shape of your face. It also sends feel-good signals to your brain.

INNER HEALTH

Improve skin condition from within by taking a cod liver oil tablet once a day. Cod liver oil is a rich source of vitamins A and D and essential fatty acids, all vital for a radiant complexion. It is also reputed to help disorders such as eczema and psoriasis.

EYE BATH

To treat puffy eyes, brew a pot of tea, leave it to cool and then use it as a soothing eye bath. Alternatively, place two stainless steel spoons in the freezer for a couple of minutes, and then place them over your eyes to reduce puffiness.

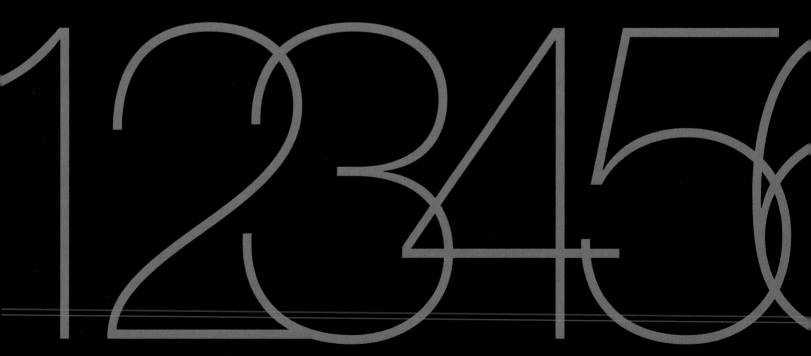

STUB IT OUT

Smoking half a packet of cigarettes a day for two years can double the rate of premature facial wrinkling. If you give up smoking, ease withdrawal symptoms by taking a high-potency vitamin B complex supplement.

HUMIDITY CONTROL

Airconditioning robs the skin of essential moisture and can aggravate dryness. If you work in an airconditioned office or use a radiator during winter, buy a humidifier or place a bowl of water next to your desk. These will boost the moisture content of the air.

HELPING HAND

If you have a youthful complexion, aged hands can give the game away. Always wear hand cream enriched with sun filters. Before washing up, slather on hand cream, then put on rubber gloves. The heat of the water will intensify the activity of the cream.

HEALTHY BREW

Research confirms that green tea can have a significant effect on the ageing process. It is a rich source of anti-oxidants, which mop up free radicals within the body. For the maximum benefit, leave the leaves or tea bags to steep for three minutes.

SLEEP WELL

How you sleep can affect your looks. Dermatologists can identify which side of your face you sleep on by looking at your wrinkles. To help overcome this, sleep on a big, soft non-synthetic pillow with a satin pillow case.

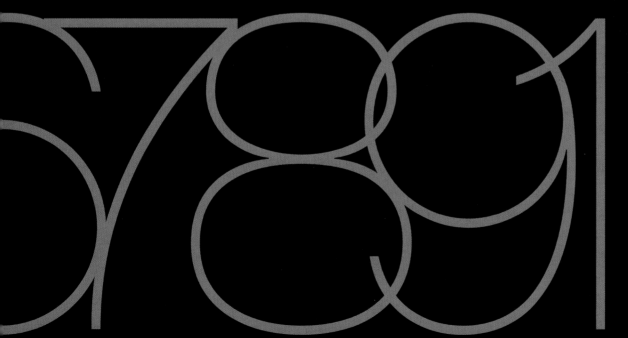

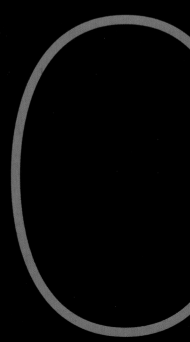

PROBLEM

How can you temporarily zap pimples?

Make-up artists use eyedrops to eradicate pimples. Dab a drop onto blemishes with a cotton bud to reduce surface redness.

Is there a way to improve problem skin?

Oily skins can be aggravated by eating certain foods. Steer clear of oranges, orange juice, tomatoes and dairy produce.

Should you wear a sunscreen every day?

Shield your skin at all times with high SPF products, even when the weather is overcast, as 60–80% of the sun's damaging ultraviolet rays penetrate clouds.

Does your skin feel taut after cleansing?

Using a harsh cleanser or rinsing with hot water can have a dehydrating effect on your skin. Use a cream cleanser to avoid this problem.

Is there a quick fix for puffy eyes?

If you wake up with puffy eyes, soak two cotton wool pads in cold milk and then use them as compresses on your eyes for 10 minutes.

Do you have **open pores?**

Often hereditary, open pores on the chin, forehead and nose can be treated with regular cleansing and facials to remove excess sebum.

How can you keep **blackheads** at bay?

Steaming your face regularly and applying face masks will treat blackheads.

How much water should you drink to maintain **healthy skin?**

Aim to drink between one and two litres of filtered or bottled spring water each day. Drinking more than this puts unnecessary pressure on the kidneys.

Should **exfoliators** be applied on wet or dry skin?

Only use an exfoliator on damp skin, otherwise it can have an abrasive effect. Avoid using an exfoliator if you have surface veins.

Do you have tiny, **pearl-coloured spots** around your eyes and cheeks?

Known as milia, these spots are formed when sebum is trapped under the skin. Seek professional help from a beauty therapist to remove them.

SOLUTION

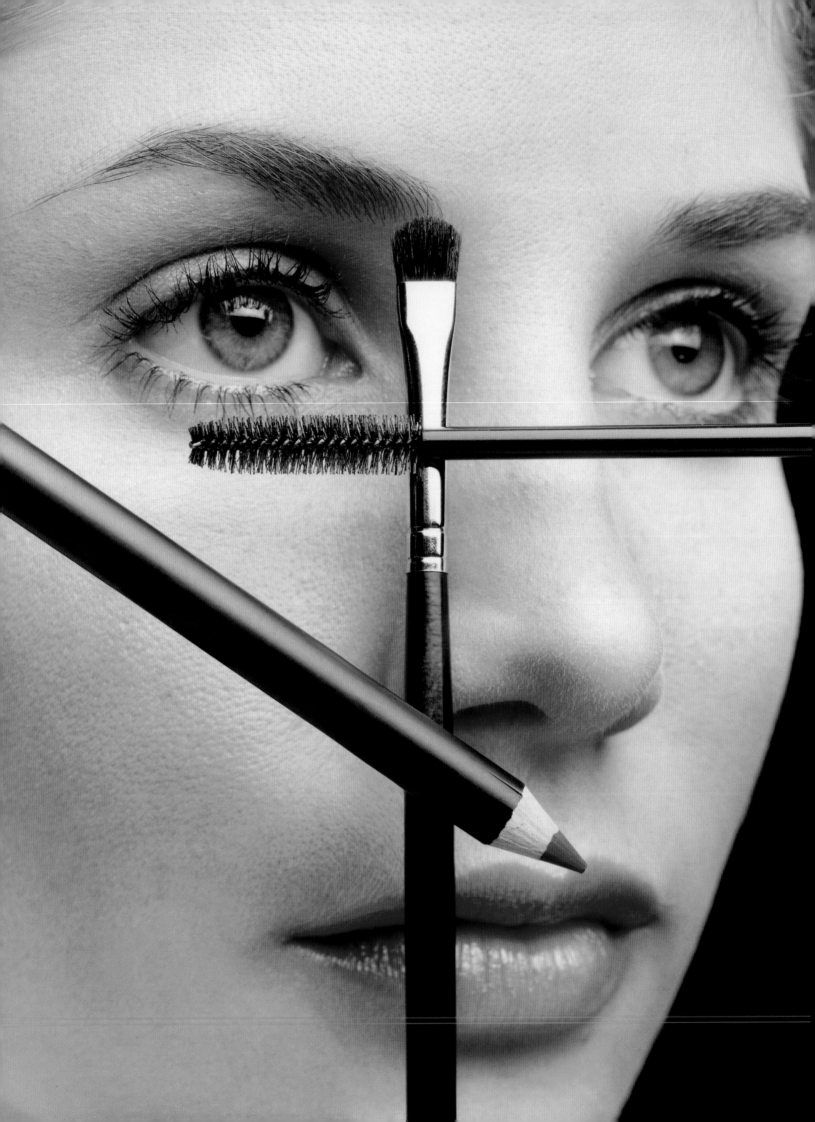

MAKE-UP

MAKE-UP SHOULD BE A TOOL TO MAKE YOU LOOK GOOD. USE COSMETICS TO ENHANCE, NOT DISGUISE, AND EXPERIMENT WITH DIFFERENT COLOURS TO ACCENTUATE YOUR NATURAL ASSETS.

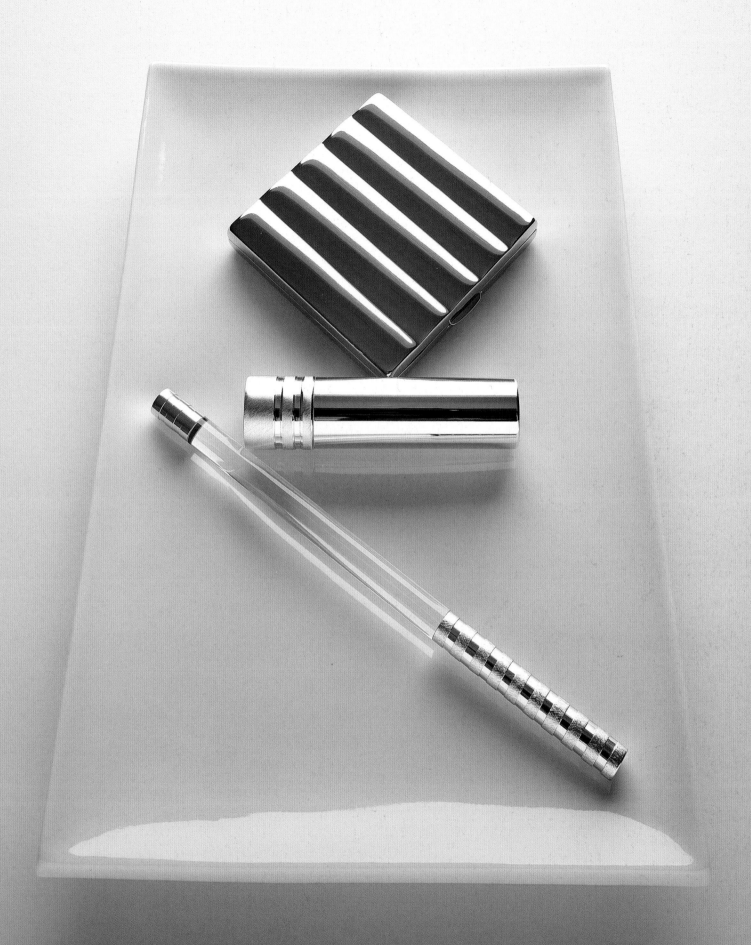

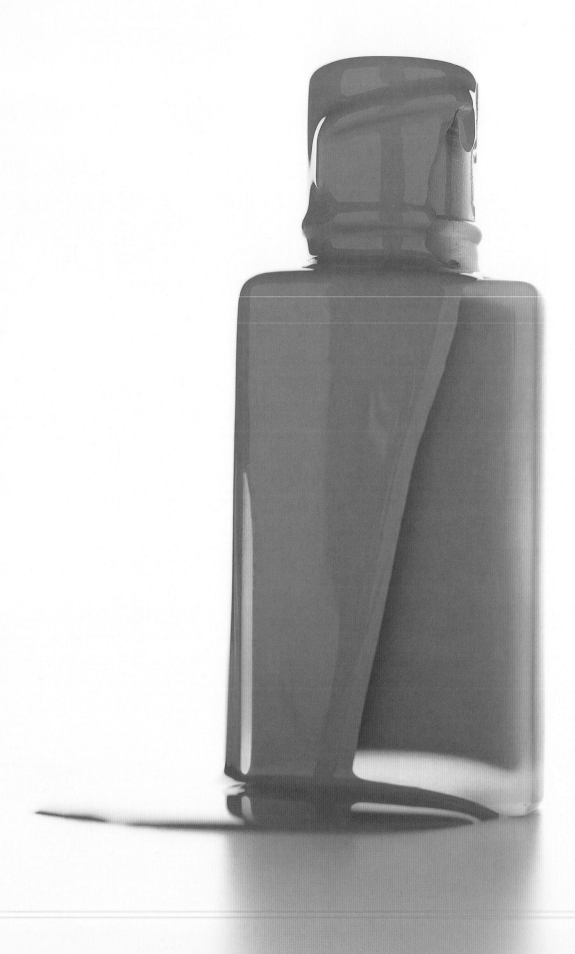

PRIMERS

Does your complexion look dull and lifeless? Do you have uneven skin tone? Are your cheeks often red? If you suffer from discolouration, spend time priming your skin to rectify problems before applying make-up. It pays off in the long run and creates the perfect canvas for cosmetic application.

COLOUR CORRECTORS work by counterbalancing their opposing hue, toning down or brightening the complexion and camouflaging imperfections. Green takes out the redness from blemishes, thread veins, ruddy cheeks and sunburn. Lilac revives tired, sallow skin and adds radiance under harsh lights. Yellow evens out skin tone and can be mixed with foundation to give the complexion a flattering finish. Blue works in harmony with pale skin, covering dark spots and toning down mild redness on the cheeks and around the base of the nose. Apricot can be used as a general pick-me-up for dull skin. White gives the skin luminosity and lightens dark circles under the eyes.

THE SECRET OF USING A COLOUR CORRECTOR lies in application and thorough blending. One of the biggest beauty blunders is a brightly coloured corrector shining through make-up. For the best results, paint the colour corrector on with a fine-tipped brush, use your fingertips to melt the colour into your skin and then apply foundation.

CONCEALER

To disguise pimples and under-eye bags, you no longer need numerous tools of the trade. An oil-free stick concealer is the best all-round option for cover-up work. Steer clear of oil-based preparations as they have a tendency to slide on and then glide off, or settle in fine lines and wrinkles. Look for a shade that is slightly lighter than your choice of foundation. If you can't find the exact colour match, try mixing a couple of shades on the back of your hand before applying.

TO DISGUISE UNDER-EYE BAGS, gently pat concealer along the orbital bone under the eye and blend it in with your fingertips. Set the area with a light dusting of powder. As signs of ageing become more obvious around the eyes, avoid using powder as it will only accentuate these traits.

TO MASK MINOR IMPERFECTIONS, use a fine-tipped make-up brush. Concentrate colour on the centre of a pimple and feather outwards. Set the area with powder. To zap blemishes, dab on a drop of lavender oil, known for its anti-bacterial properties, under concealer. If camouflaged imperfections dry out and look unsightly during the day, pat on a little moisturiser with your fingertip and lightly dust with powder. This instantly gives the skin a new lease of life.

LIQUID FOUNDATIONS

come in various forms. Water-based
formulas suit combination or problem skins;
oil-based formulas help hydrate dry skins;
and oil-free variants are ideal for oily skins.

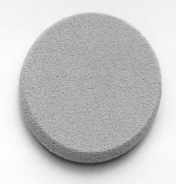

COMPACT FOUNDATIONS

combine foundation and powder in
one and are easy to use. This type of
foundation is suitable for all skin types.

STICK FOUNDATIONS

provide excellent coverage but can be
difficult to apply. Smooth on with your
fingertips or use a damp sponge.

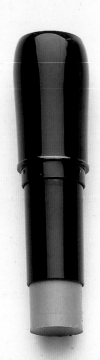

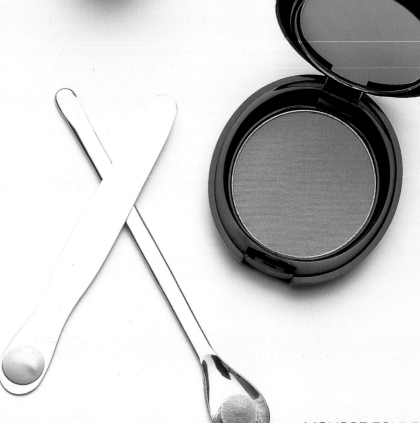

TINTED MOISTURISERS

both enhance and provide protection
from the sun. However, shades are
limited and coverage is minimal. They
are great for summer wear.

MOUSSE FOUNDATIONS

are light and airy and feel weightless once
applied. As coverage is minimal, they suit
young, blemish-free skins.

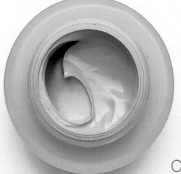

CREAM FORMULATIONS

have a moisture-rich feel, which makes
them perfect for dry skins. They give extra
coverage and provide a dewy finish.

FOUNDATION

Foundation should cover but not whitewash your entire face. With clever application, foundation can mask imperfections and at the same time give your skin a clean, seemingly unmade-up finish.

SHADE SELECTION

Finding the perfect colour match is one of the toughest beauty jobs and it can make or break your look.

EXPERIMENT WITH DIFFERENT SHADES and take into account your natural skin tone. Fair complexions should opt for ivory bases with yellow undertones and steer clear of pinkish shades. Yellow-toned complexions should go for a beige base with a yellow undertone. Olive skins need pinkish-toned foundation, otherwise the skin will look sallow and dull. Dark complexions often suffer from uneven skin tone, so use foundation to rectify this. Opt for a shade that is specifically formulated for dark skin, otherwise the complexion will appear ashy from the excess of titanium dioxide contained in most products. Consider whether your skin is dry, normal or oily and find the right formulation to suit your skin type.

APPLICATION

Use foundation sparingly and only apply it where necessary (to the T-zone or to camouflage imperfections). Complete foundation coverage can make your face appear caked and unnatural.

FOR THE BEST RESULTS, warm foundation on the back of your hand and then smooth it on with your fingertips. Apply compact foundations with a damp or dry sponge, depending on the desired result. For maximum coverage, use a damp sponge but work quickly because the formula dries fast. For retouches, apply foundation with a dry sponge.

POWDER

Powder is the perfect tool to set your base and keep any oily secretions at bay. The choice of pressed or loose powder depends on personal preference. Pressed formulations are easy to use and ideal for retouches, while loose powders can be messy to apply.

USE FACE POWDER ONLY WHERE ESSENTIAL. Dust it onto areas prone to shine such as the nose, chin and forehead. For the best results, use a large brush and work down your face (to prevent particles of powder from catching under superfluous facial hair and giving an uneven finish). Always blow on a loaded brush before dusting on powder. This removes excess powder and prevents overload. After applying powder, set your base by spritzing your face with mineral water or facial toner. This ensures a fresh, dewy finish that does not look too powdered.

TRICKS OF THE TRADE

To test foundation shades, select three appropriate colours and put a streak of each over your face and jawline. The foundation that literally disappears into the skin is the appropriate one. Never sample shades on the back of your hand as the skin there is a different tone to the skin on your face.

If you have sensitive skin, avoid foundations containing fragrance and PABA sunscreens.

Foundation can slide off within hours of application because of the skin's natural oil secretions. To solve this, use a formula incorporating oil absorbers such as talc, kaolin or nylon powders.

Shield your skin with a foundation containing a sun-protection factor. This is essential for daily wear, even when the weather is overcast.

Blot your skin with a tissue after applying foundation to remove excess oil from your face. This helps to prolong the life of your make-up base. Then set with powder.

Wash sponges, powder puffs or special applicators regularly. Use warm water and a little dishwashing liquid to remove bacteria and impurities.

EYEBROWS

Eyebrows act as a frame for your eyes and add definition and strength to your face. Even if you are not wearing make-up, well-groomed eyebrows enhance your total look.

TO SHAPE YOUR EYEBROWS, invest in a pair of slant-edged tweezers which grip hairs easily. Pluck before going to bed, so if the skin is a little red it will calm down while you sleep. Use your facial features as a guideline to shape your eyebrows. Place a ruler or pencil vertically alongside your nose and the inner edge of each eye. This is where the brows should start. Swivel the ruler or pencil from the top to the outer corner of the eye. This is where the brows should end.

BEFORE PLUCKING, comb the brows one way and then the other to remove any loose hairs and then brush them into shape. Pluck hairs between the brows and any stragglers but never remove hairs from above your eyebrows. To achieve the perfect arch, hold a ruler vertically next to the outside of the iris – this should be the central point of the arch. Pull the skin taut and pluck hairs individually, grasping close to the root, always working in the direction of growth. To avoid over-plucking, make-up artists recommend drawing in the desired brow shape with a pale concealer and using this as a guideline.

TO DEFINE YOUR EYEBROWS, use a shade similar to your natural hair colour and aim for an unmade-up looking finish. If you use a pencil, apply in small, feathered strokes (no longer than the average brow hair). Start at the inner corner of the brow and work outwards, then blend the colour with a brush or your fingertips. Alternatively, use a sponge-tipped applicator and dust on a natural shade of eyeshadow that complements your hair colour, and follow the shape of the brow.

TO TAME UNRULY EYEBROWS and keep stray hairs in place, don't splash out on expensive products. Slick moisturiser, hair gel or lip gloss through your brows and comb through to neaten them. Instead of discarding old mascara wands, clean them thoroughly with soap and warm water and then use them as brow-grooming implements.

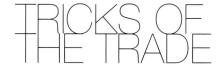

TRICKS OF THE TRADE

Sharpen blunt tweezers by running sandpaper over the inner tips.

If plucking is too painful, smooth on baby's teething gel to temporarily numb the area.

Substitute a toothbrush for a brow comb to groom your brows.

If you are slapdash when applying brow pencil, take a tip from the experts. Rub the pencil on the back of your hand. Run over the mark you've made with a brow brush or cotton bud and use this to shade the brows instead.

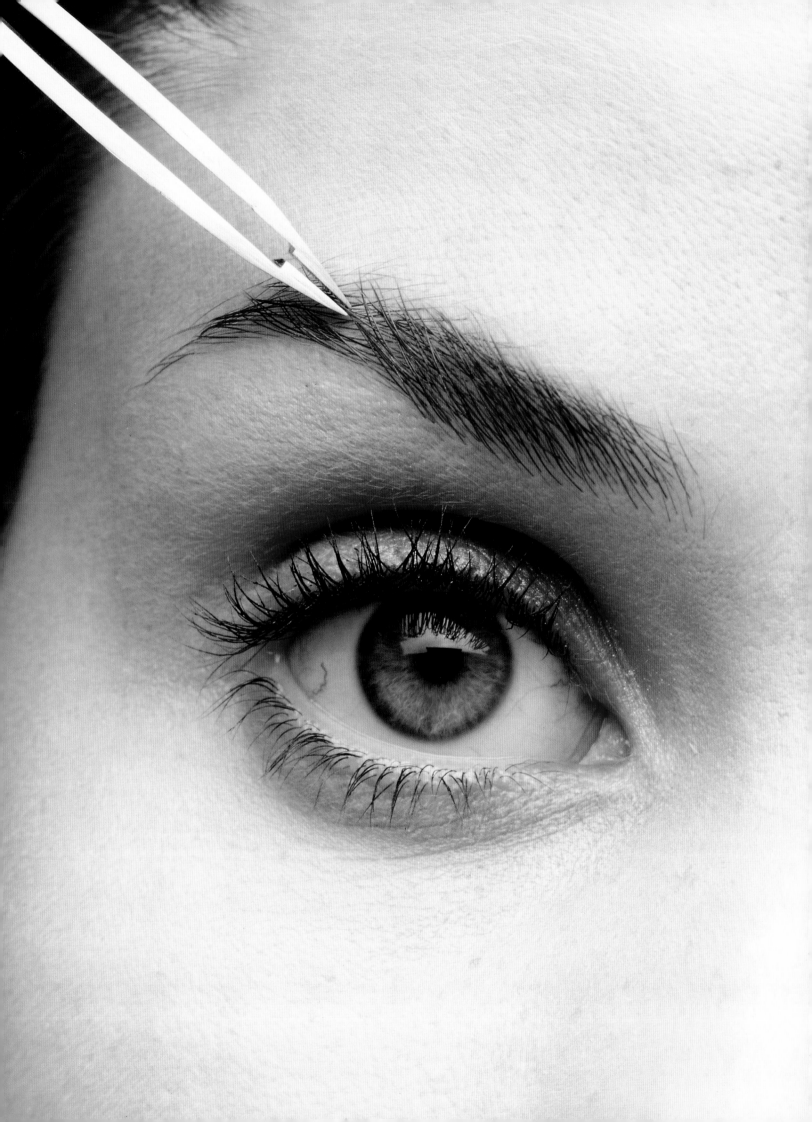

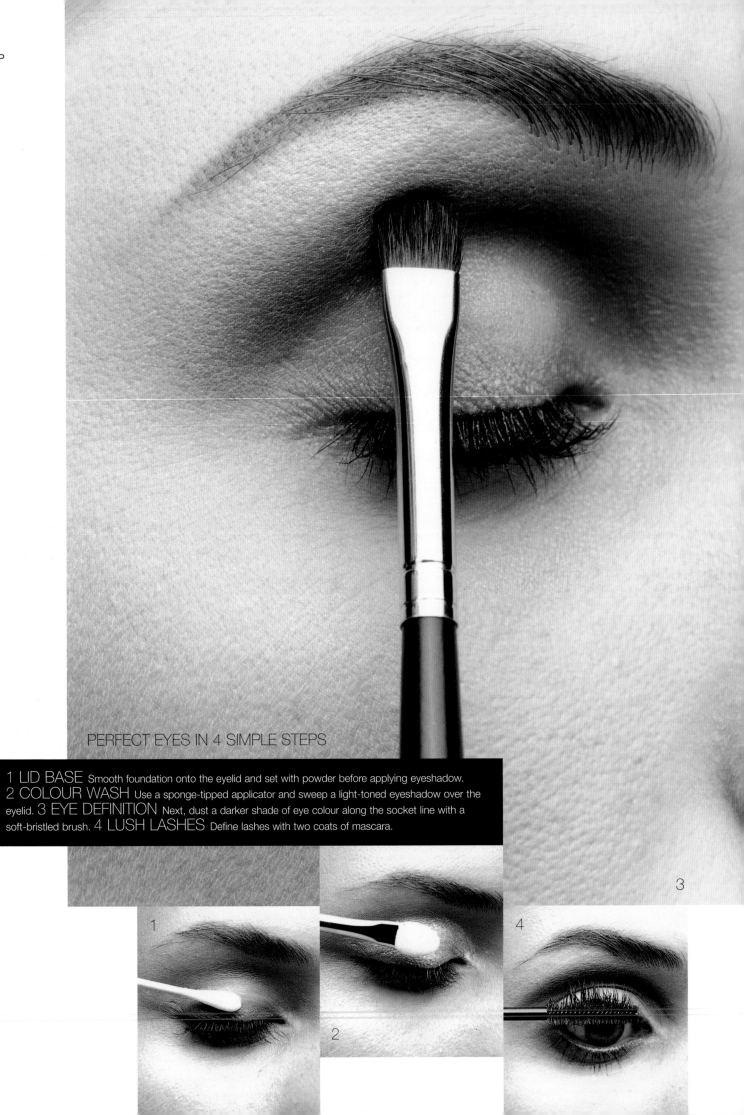

PERFECT EYES IN 4 SIMPLE STEPS

1 LID BASE Smooth foundation onto the eyelid and set with powder before applying eyeshadow.
2 COLOUR WASH Use a sponge-tipped applicator and sweep a light-toned eyeshadow over the eyelid. **3 EYE DEFINITION** Next, dust a darker shade of eye colour along the socket line with a soft-bristled brush. **4 LUSH LASHES** Define lashes with two coats of mascara.

EYESHADOW

Use eyeshadow to shade and highlight your eyes. Once you have mastered the basics of application, experiment with colour. Remember that shades are not nearly as intense as they appear in their palettes – always apply them sparingly and gradually build up colour. Never match eyeshadow with the colour of your iris – look for shades that will enhance and bring out the natural hue of your eyes. As you age, it's best to avoid wearing pearlised eyeshadows; matt colours have a more flattering effect on mature eyes.

TO ACHIEVE A WEARABLE FINISH, use a natural shade as a wash over the eyelid. For swift application, sweep a cotton ball over eyeshadow and gently dust it on in one stroke. For more definition, apply a deeper shade of the colour along the lash line or shade it into the eye socket. If you're pushed for time, just dab a hint of colour onto the centre of the eyelid and blend it outwards using your fingertips. If you prefer not to wear eyeshadow, you can always add subtle touches of colour using pencils and mascaras.

EYELINER

Use eyeliner to define and enhance your eyes. Pencils are easy to use and you don't need to be a professional to apply them. Should uneven lines or mishaps occur, simply smudge them into shape with a sponge-tipped applicator. Liquid eyeliner is the perfect tool to give eyes instant glamour but it can be tricky to apply. To make the task easier, place a mirror flat on a table and rest the hand manoeuvring the liner on this hard surface. Look down into the mirror and apply the liner. To improve the staying power of eyeliner, dip a moistened cotton bud into a similar shade of eyeshadow and use this to trace the line.

MASCARA

Before applying mascara, always give the lashes a quick fix with lash curlers. Clamp them near the roots and hold for 30 seconds. Never curl lashes loaded with mascara – you run the risk of tearing them from the roots if the mascara dries or catches on the curlers.

TO INSTANTLY PLUMP UP LASHES, plant the mascara wand into the root and sweep through to the tips. This gives root definition and separates the lashes at the same time. To define your lower lashes, use the tip of the wand and gently work the brush horizontally over the lashes. Separate the lashes using a comb and rectify any mishaps with a cotton bud.

TRICKS OF THE TRADE

If your eye pencil crumbles as you're using it, clasp the nib between your fingers and run it under cold water. This temporarily hardens the pencil to ease application.

Use a white eyeliner to define the inner rim of the lower lash line. This instantly opens your eyes and makes the whites appear brighter.

If you are short-sighted, corrective lenses will magnify your eyes. Opt for eyeshadows in muted colours.

If you are far-sighted, glasses make your eyes appear smaller. Go for brighter eyeshadow and several coats of mascara to make your eyes stand out.

If you have close-set eyes, concentrate light colours on the inner corners and darker shades on the outer edges of your eyes.

To lift droopy eyes, shade the outer corners of the eyes, tapering colour upwards and outwards.

To elongate round eyes, use colour on the mid and outer eyelid. Don't apply eyeliner on the lower lash line.

If you have wide-set eyes, use darker colours on the inner corners and light shades on the outer edges of your eyes.

To enhance small eyes, avoid using dark eyeshadow and concentrate colour on the socket lines and outer corners of your eyes.

TRICKS OF THE TRADE

Protect your lips with lip balm or lipstick containing SPF 15. The lips do not contain melanin, the body's natural sun-defence substance, and the lower lip is a common site for skin cancers.

If you're in a hurry, avoid wearing red and dark-coloured lipsticks as they require precision application. Try lipsticks with neutral tones.

Avoid dark lip colours if you have narrow lips. Paler shades enhance the shape of the lips, making them appear fuller.

To enhance a pout, dab silver lip gloss onto the centre of the lower lip.

If your lip liner is too dark and won't work in harmony with your chosen lip colour, tone it down with a small amount of foundation, then apply lipstick.

Give your lips a top coat of vitamin E oil. It seals in the colour, creates instant shine and helps to condition and protect this sensitive area.

Brightly coloured lipsticks look great but there's a catch: because of the density of their colour pigment, they tend to feather and bleed around the lip-line. To prevent this, define and coat the lips with liner before applying lipstick.

There is nothing more taboo than lipstick on your teeth. To prevent this, put your index finger in your mouth and close your lips. As you withdraw your finger it will remove any excess colour which could end up on your teeth.

LIP LINER

Lip liner accentuates the shape of the lips. Invest in a pencil that is close to your lips' natural colour and team this with any shade of lipstick. It can be tricky to achieve the perfect lip-line, especially if you are a little over-enthusiastic and don't have a steady hand. The best method is to apply the liner in a series of feather-strokes around the outer edge of the lips, then join and blend these with your fingertips or a lip brush.

USE LIP LINER TO DEFINE AND SHADE the entire lip area. Otherwise, when the lipstick wears off, you'll be left with an unsightly outline. Lip liner also acts as a fixative for lipstick.

IF YOU WANT TO DO CORRECTIVE WORK, for example, plump up narrow lips or emphasise a cupid's bow, keep it to a minimum. It can look messy and require constant retouches. Instead, experiment with different shades of lipstick. Pale tones add fullness to the lips and dark shades have a slimming effect.

LIP GLOSS

Lip gloss, available in clear or tinted versions, is ideal for highlighting your lips or enhancing your mouth's natural colour. Because of its consistency, it tends to slide on and glide off within hours of application, or seeps into fine lines around the mouth. To overcome this, dab gloss onto the centre of the upper and lower lip, and then purse your lips together. This creates the illusion of all-over gloss.

LIPSTICK

You don't have to match your lipstick with your clothing or nail varnish. For a modern finish, take your skin tone and overall make-up look into consideration. Shades with brown undertones will flatter most complexions.

THERE IS A GREAT VARIETY OF LIPSTICK TEXTURES, which range from matt and cream to sheer tints. Experiment with these, bearing in mind that matt is long-lasting but has a tendency to dehydrate the lips; creamy formulations last well; and lip tints provide a natural look and add lustre.

APPLICATION

The way you apply lipstick is up to you. Experiment with brushes and your fingertips and see what you feel comfortable with. To improve the staying power of lipstick, blot the lips with a tissue after application and reapply. Repeat this several times. Add a final coat of lipstick. Alternatively, once you've applied lipstick, place a tissue over the lips and dust them with a small amount of loose powder, then remove the tissue.

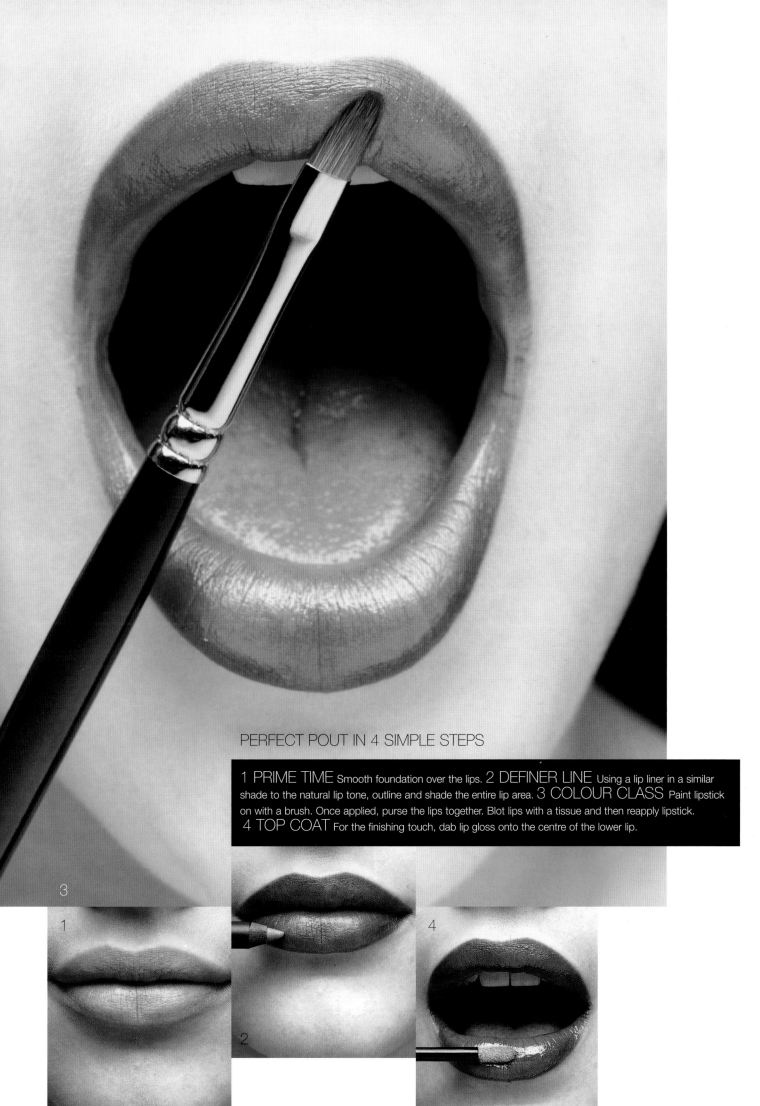

PERFECT POUT IN 4 SIMPLE STEPS

1 PRIME TIME Smooth foundation over the lips. 2 DEFINER LINE Using a lip liner in a similar shade to the natural lip tone, outline and shade the entire lip area. 3 COLOUR CLASS Paint lipstick on with a brush. Once applied, purse the lips together. Blot lips with a tissue and then reapply lipstick. 4 TOP COAT For the finishing touch, dab lip gloss onto the centre of the lower lip.

Create your own blusher
by using a natural pink or apricot shade of lipstick and dab it onto your cheek apples. Blend thoroughly using your fingertips.

To fade a double chin,
blend a shader onto the area to make it less dominant. If you darken the double chin, it will recede into the background.

Use creamy eyeshadow
in natural shades if you've run out of cream blusher.

To transform daytime blush
into evening glamour, dust a shimmery gold powder over the top of the blusher.

To add a healthy glow,
employ a bronzing powder as a blusher and gradually build up the colour.

For a flattering finish if you
don't wear eyeshadow, sweep blusher over your eyelids to give subtle definition.

BLUSHER

Blusher should be used to add the finishing touches to your make-up and also to warm your skin. Whether you use a cream or powder formulation, the aim is to give your cheeks subtle definition and balance your total cosmetic look.

CREAM BLUSHERS are easy to apply as they literally melt into the skin. They're also beneficial for older skins as they won't accentuate fine lines and wrinkles. Powder blushers are also easy to use and can be applied in seconds. Use your foundation finish as a guideline to choose a blusher formulation: team powdered complexions with powder blusher and creamy bases with cream blusher. Choose a shade that complements your make-up and skin tone. Use your lipstick colour as a guide or invest in a natural tone which will flatter your skin and work well with any make-up look.

APPLICATION

Be careful not to place the colour too close to the outer corners of your eyes when you apply blusher. It can creep into lines and crow's-feet around the eyes and look caked. Also, always ensure you blend blusher thoroughly.

TO CONTOUR YOUR CHEEKS, use a brush and follow the line of your cheekbone, working in small, circular movements. Dust the blusher on from the top of the bone downwards so that the colour fade is gradual.

TO GIVE YOUR CHEEKS A ROSY GLOW, concentrate blusher onto the cheek apples, the roundest part of the cheekbone. Dust the colour on the centre of the bone and work in small circular motions to achieve a natural finish.

CHANGING FACES

You can temporarily transform the shape of your face with a shader (a tone deeper than your existing blusher) and a high-lighter (you can use an ivory-coloured eyeshadow). Use these lightly and blend thoroughly.

ROUND FACES Dust shader into your cheek hollows, high on your temples next to your hairline and faintly under your chin. Highlight along your cheekbones. Wearing blusher is optional but be wary of dusting it onto your cheek apples – this may emphasise the roundness of your face.

OVAL FACES Blend shader into cheek hollows and highlight the cheekbones near your eyes. Dust blusher onto cheek apples.

HEART-SHAPED FACES To balance your face, highlight your chin, shade your temples and dust blusher into your cheek hollows.

SQUARE FACES Highlight the central strip from the centre of your forehead to your chin. Shade the sides of your forehead next to your hairline and faintly shade the square extremities of your jawline. Dust blusher onto your cheek apples.

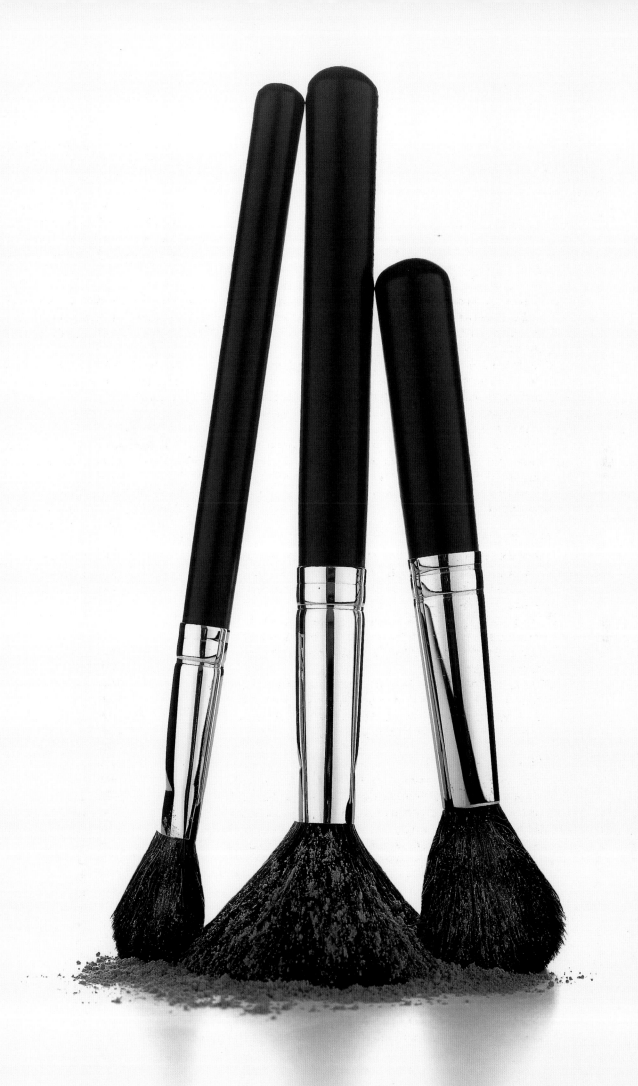

PERFECT POLISH IN 4 SIMPLE STEPS

1 BASE COAT Apply a fast-drying base coat, ensuring it goes on thinly to provide an even surface for polish. Leave to dry for 60 seconds. 2 FINE LINE Always apply polish in three strokes (down the centre of the nail and then one on either side). Leave a tiny margin free around the cuticle to achieve a professional finish. 3 TOP COAT Paint on a top coat to protect the nails. 4 FINISHING TOUCH When the nail polish is touch-dry, run your fingertips under cold water to help set the polish thoroughly.

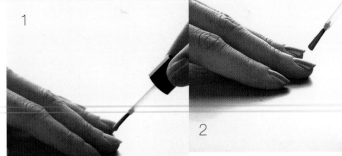

NAIL POLISH

Whether you opt for a pale enamel or the fashionable colour of the moment, nail polish can accentuate your hands and add the finishing touches to your complete beauty look.

WHEN SELECTING SHADES OF NAIL ENAMEL, take your skin tone into account. Use the inside of your wrist as a guideline. If your skin has a bluish tinge, opt for shades with a cool base. If you have yellow- or olive-toned skin, opt for a warm-based polish. Avoid co-ordinating the colour of your fingernails and toenails and never fall into the trap of matching nail polish with clothing and lipstick. A mismatched look is much more modern.

EXPRESS MANICURE

To keep your nails in optimum condition, run a soft-bristled nailbrush horizontally over them whilst in the shower. This will treat the cuticles, step up circulation and strengthen your nails.

FORGET PUSHING THE CUTICLES BACK MANUALLY. Look for a cuticle cream enriched with an alpha hydroxy acid complex. It helps dissolve dead skin cells and keeps cuticles in order.

REMOVE OLD POLISH WITH AN ACETONE POLISH. It will temporarily dehydrate the nails so polish locks onto the nail plate more effectively.

TAKE SHORT CUTS TO SHAPE YOUR NAILS. Use nail clippers first, then finish with a nail file. Only work the file in one direction otherwise you can traumatise the nail plate.

THE SECRET TO A LASTING MANICURE lies in preparation. Before applying polish, run your hands under warm water and wash with a lanolin-free soap to remove any residues of nail treatments which can weaken nail polish. Your nails will then be ready for the application of colour.

TRICKS OF THE TRADE

Nails need protection from the sun. Use a top coat enriched with UV filters. This also protects the nail polish from discolouration.

Never trim your cuticles. They protect the nail bed and act as a barrier against intruding bacteria. Gently push the cuticles back with a wet facecloth whilst in the shower.

If you have uneven ridges in your nails, avoid pearly or frosted polishes as they highlight imperfections.

To make nail polish last, store it in the fridge. To ensure an even consistency, never shake a bottle of nail polish. Instead, turn it upside down once and then gently roll it between the palms of your hands.

If you're pushed for time, give nude nails a high shine by running a chamois buffer over them in horizontal sweeping motions.

Invest in specialty products such as base coat and top coat as they have different purposes. A base coat feels sticky once applied to act as a fixative for nail enamel. It also prevents dark-coloured polishes from staining the nail plate. A top coat dries hard, locking in colour to give the surface a hard, protective barrier.

To clean up any smudges and imperfections, use an old, clean lip brush dipped in nail polish remover.

If the nail plate is stained from wearing highly pigmented polish, dissolve two denture-cleansing tablets in a glass of water. Dip a nail brush into the solution and gently scrub your nails clean. Rinse your hands with warm water.

TOOLS OF THE TRADE

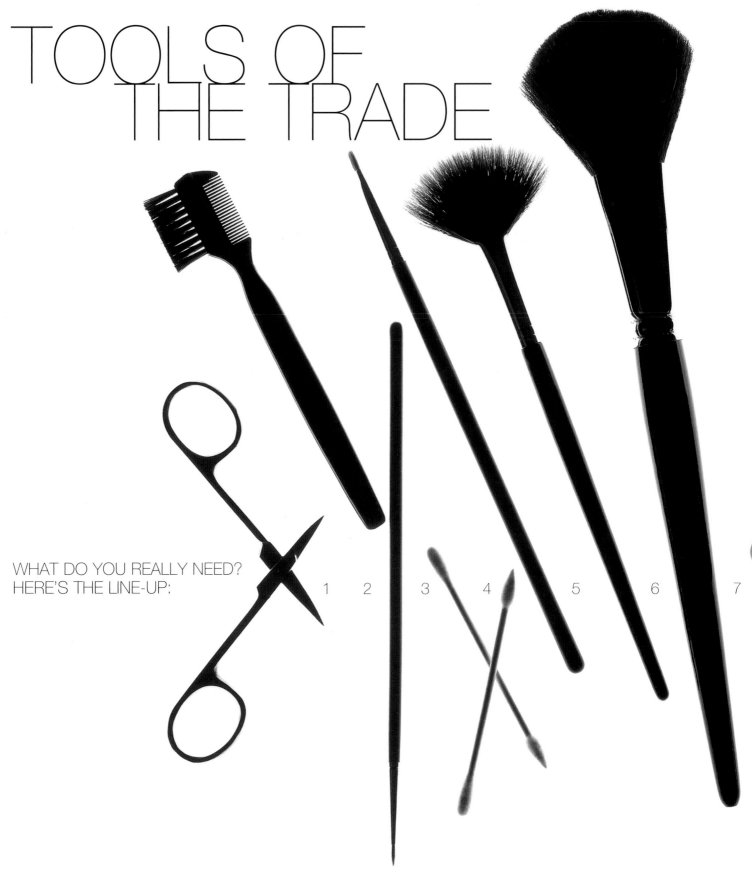

WHAT DO YOU REALLY NEED?
HERE'S THE LINE-UP:

1   2   3   4   5   6   7

1 SCISSORS An essential tool for beauty up-keep. 2 EYEBROW TAMER/LASH COMB Use the brush to tame eyebrows and the comb to separate eyelashes. 3 FINE-TIPPED BRUSH To conceal pimples and minor imperfections. 4 COTTON BUDS Essential to rectify make-up mistakes. 5 LIP BRUSH Use to outline and shade lips. 6 FLAT BRUSH This is a must to remove stray particles of eyeshadow which can fall under the eyes during application. 7 POWDER BRUSH A large-bristled brush delivers just the right amount of powder. 8 BLUSHER BRUSH Use this brush to dust colour gently onto the cheek apples or to accentuate the shape of the cheekbones.

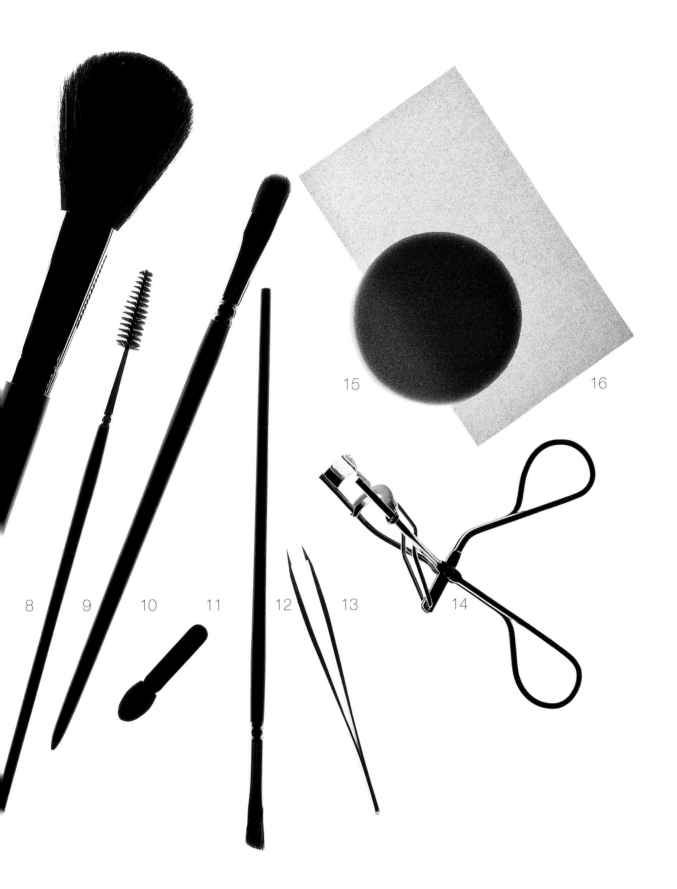

8   9   10   11   12   13   14

15   16

9 LASH GROOMER To tidy lashes and define their shape, especially if you're not wearing mascara. 10 EYESHADOW BRUSH A soft-bristled brush is ideal for blending eyeshadow and defining the eye socket with colour. 11 SPONGE-TIPPED APPLICATOR For applying eyeshadow. 12 SLANT-EDGED BRUSH Perfect for shading the brows with eyeshadow. 13 TWEEZERS Slant-edged tweezers grab hold of the hairs to ease plucking. 14 EYELASH CURLERS Giving the lashes definition instantly opens the eyes. 15 SPONGE Use to smooth on foundation and to set your base after application. 16 TISSUES A necessity for blotting foundation and lipstick after applying.

EXPRESS MAKE-OVER

FOLLOW THESE STEPS TO ACHIEVE A NATURAL LOOK

PRIME TIME

Begin by applying a hydrating preparation to give your skin a smooth finish. This will also act as the perfect fixative for foundation. Always blot your skin with a tissue after moisturising to remove any excess surface oil.

TAKE COVER

Conceal pimples and disguise imperfections. To touch out blemishes, apply concealer with a fine-tipped brush. Dab colour onto the centre of the pimple, then feather outwards. Pat concealer under the eyes, blending with the fingertips.

TOUCH BASE

Use a foundation with a built-in sunscreen. Smooth it on with your fingertips, warming it to melt into your skin. Only apply to areas that need it, where the skin tone is uneven, or to disguise open pores. Blend thoroughly.

PERFECT POWDER

Keep powder to a minimum. Look for a yellow-undertoned formula as translucent powder zaps colour and may leave you looking washed out. Only dust powder onto areas prone to shine like the nose and chin.

BRIGHT EYES

Dab a light-toned eye-shadow onto the eyelid using a sponge-tipped applicator. Then apply a darker shade of the same colour on the socket line with an eye-shadow brush. Blend thoroughly to achieve gradual colour change.

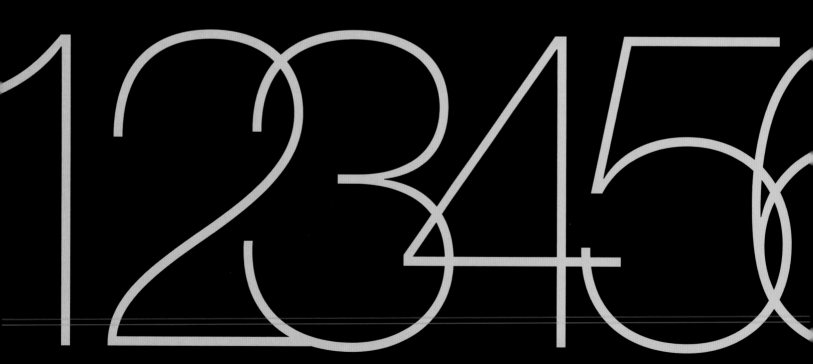

DEFINER LINE

Define the lower lash line with a taupe kohl pencil, then set with a light dusting of eye-shadow (the same shade used on the eye socket). Applying liner on the upper lash line isn't necessary to achieve a natural look.

MAGIC WAND

Enhance your eyelashes by gradually plumping them up with several coats of mascara. This will be far more flattering than making one heavy-handed application. Plant the wand into the roots and gently pull through to the ends.

COLOUR WASH

Use a lip liner in a shade that is similar to the natural colour of your lips. Outline and shade the entire lip area. Next, apply a reddish brown lipstick and blot with a tissue. Reapply and repeat this process several times.

BLUSH TACTIC

To give your cheeks subtle colour, load a blusher brush with a rosy beige powder, gently blow on it to remove excess powder, then softly sculpt the cheekbones. Set by pressing a damp sponge into the skin.

TOP COAT

Add the final touches with a slick of clear lip gloss. To accentuate your pout, concentrate shine on the centre of the lower lip. To define your eyebrows, smooth them into place with a small amount of gloss and comb to neaten.

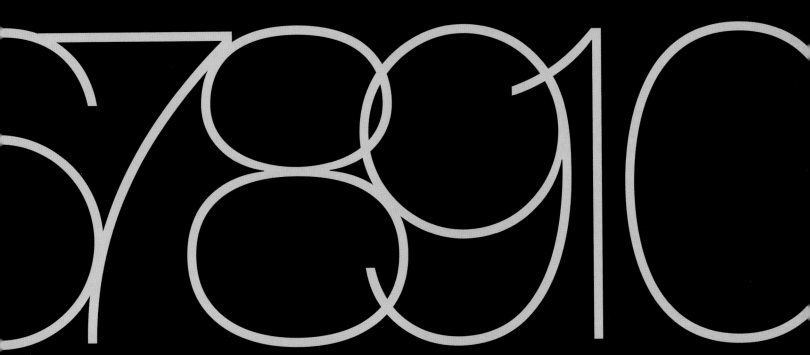

PROBLEM

Does your blusher **vanish within hours of application?**
Overcome this with double-colour application. Pat on cream blusher over foundation and then set with powder blusher in a similar shade.

Do you end up with mascara-clogged lashes?
Prior to application, wipe the mascara wand with a tissue. This removes the excess mascara which can overload the eyelashes.

Does your foundation **emphasise fine lines and wrinkles?**
Avoid wearing matt foundations – they will only accentuate lines and wrinkles. Creamy formulas give a dewy finish and detract from signs of ageing.

Do you suffer from tired, lifeless-looking eyes?
Applying a smudge of silver shine on the inner corner of each eye will instantly revitalise and brighten sleepy-looking eyes.

Do you find it tricky to apply eyeliner?
Dot eyeliner along the lash lines and use a fine-tipped brush to join the dots. This is the easiest and most effective way to achieve a straight line.

Can you achieve great-looking nails in a hurry?
Run a white eyeliner underneath the nail tip and then paint the nails with a fast-drying coat of clear polish. This creates a French-manicured effect within minutes.

How do you remove traces of smudged eyeliner or flaky mascara without disturbing the rest of your make-up?
Arm yourself with cotton buds or an old, clean lip brush. Dip the bud or brush in make-up remover and gently use it to perfect mistakes.

Are you too heavy-handed with blusher?
Tone down unsightly colour by pressing face powder into your cheeks, then spritz your skin with water or facial toner.

Do you look artificial once you've applied your make-up?
Gently press a damp cosmetic sponge onto your face, it will transform a powdered finish into fresh-faced beauty.

Is your lip pencil hard to manoeuvre?
Gently run the nib of the pencil over the back of the hand before applying.

SOLUTION

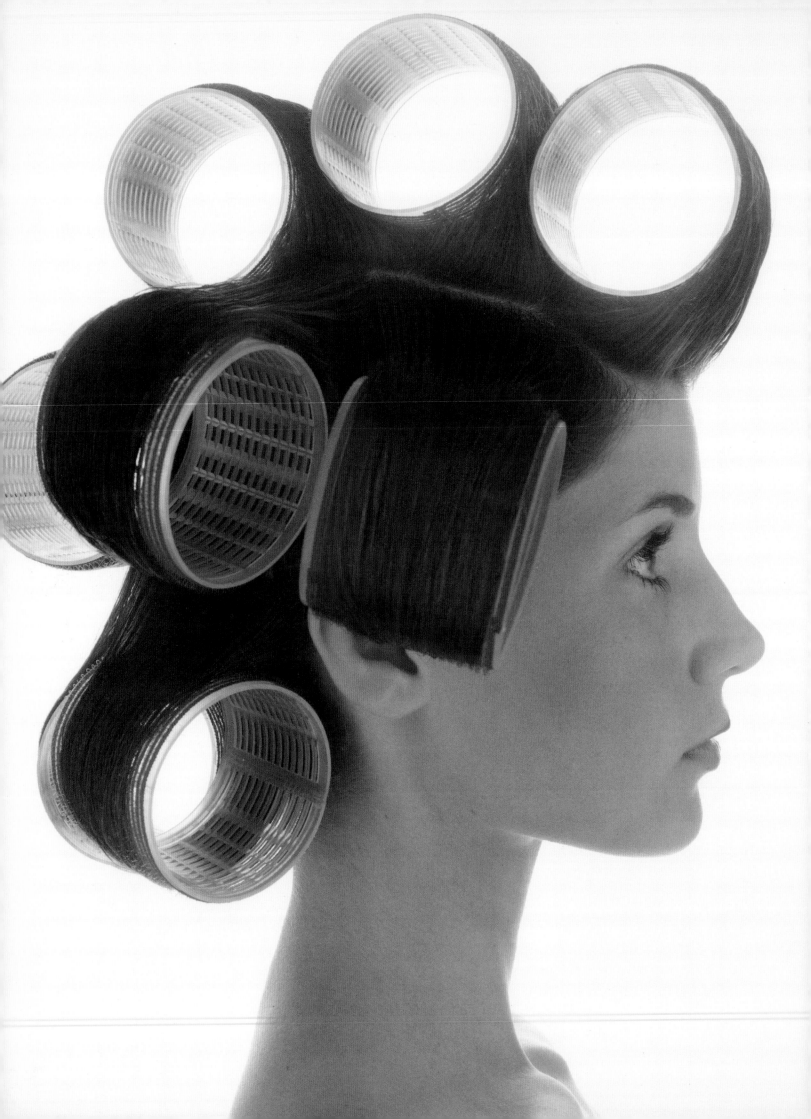

HAIR

Hair is a barometer of your inner health. The secret to lustrous locks lies in the cut, condition and colour. Banish bad hair days and make hair your crowning glory.

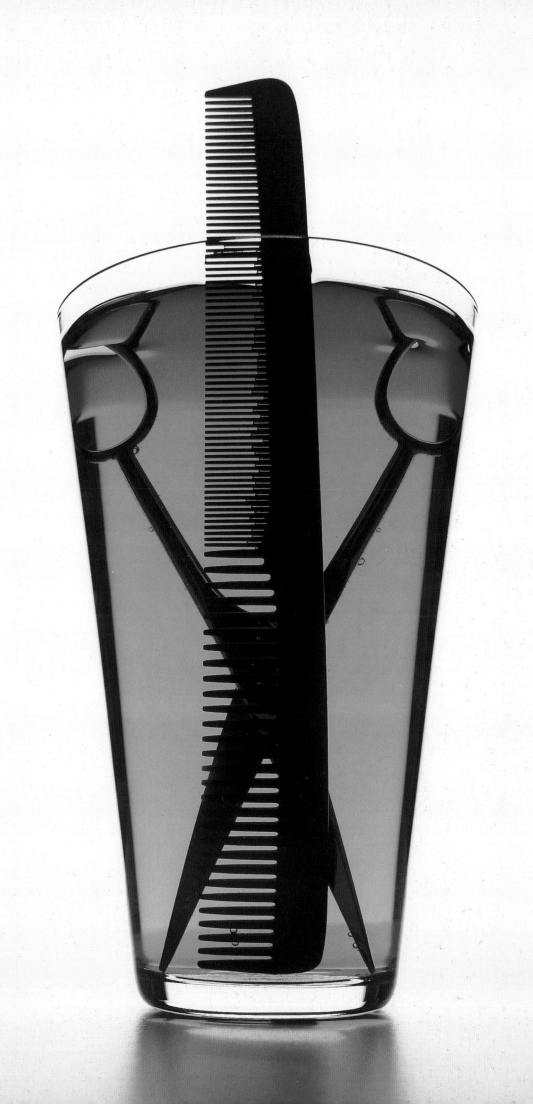

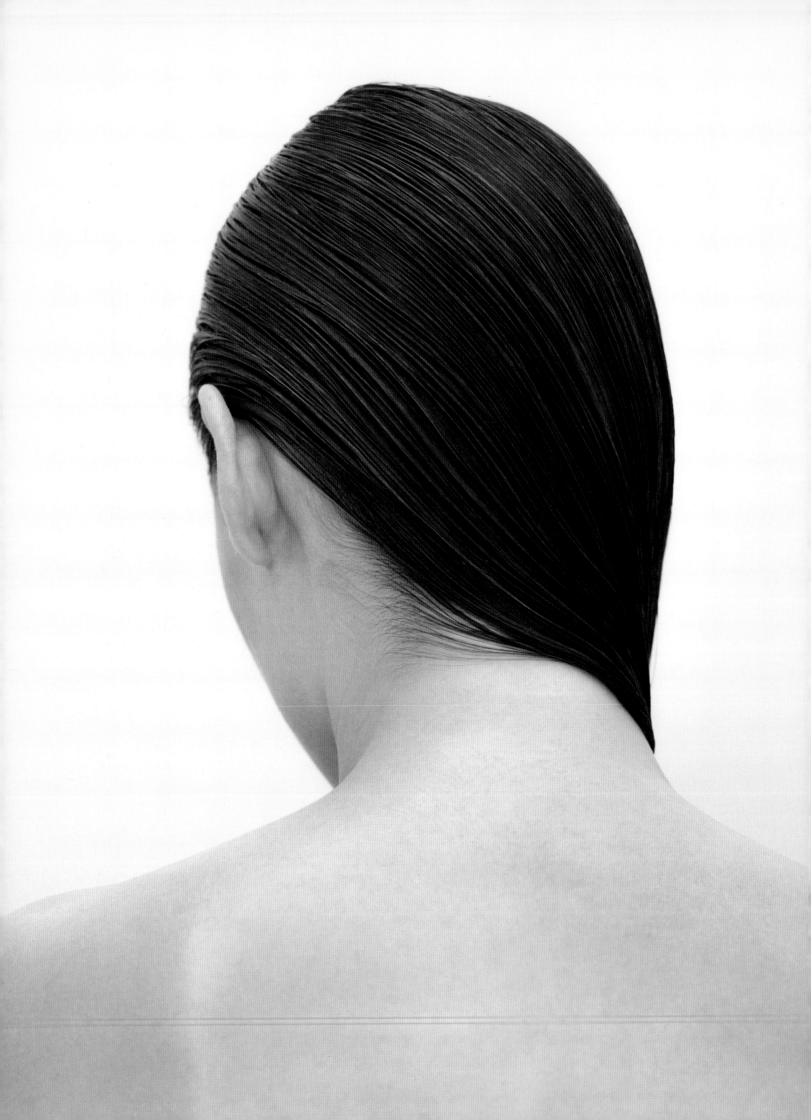

HAIRCARE

The condition of your hair, just like that of your skin, is determined by your inner health. The stresses and strains of modern living can take their toll – lacklustre locks probably mean that your body is not functioning as it should be. Achieve healthy-looking locks with a nutritious diet and an effective maintenance regime. First identify your hair type and then choose a haircare regime accordingly.

NORMAL HAIR is often a result of genetic good fortune. If you are blessed with this hair type, look after it. A basic haircare regime is sufficient, and taking a multivitamin daily will maintain hair health. Avoid harsh haircare products, exposure to the sun and heated styling appliances.

GREASY HAIR is usually the result of hormonal imbalances, poor diet, stress and harsh haircare products. Characterised by an oily scalp and dry ends, this condition is caused by over-active sebaceous glands, which produce excess amounts of sebum (the hair's natural lubricating oil).

DRY HAIR is caused by factors including poor nutrition, chemical treatments (such as colouring or perming), exposure to the sun, and the use of heated styling appliances. This hair type doesn't receive enough sebum, which makes it coarse and brittle and susceptible to damage.

BRUSHING

When you select grooming implements, take into account both your hair texture and your styling requirements. Natural bristle brushes, which are made of keratin (the same material as hair), are the least damaging, but the bristles are too soft to benefit thick hair. A combination of natural and synthetic bristles is effective for thicker hair. For curly hair, brushes with closely spaced, all-synthetic bristles offer maximum control.

FOR STYLING, a flat brush is best for general maintenance and to smooth and detangle the hair, while a round brush will help add volume and curl or straighten locks as you're blow-drying. Vent brushes are ideal for blow-drying if you're in a hurry – the vents in the brush enable the air from the dryer to circulate freely through both the brush and the hair, making it dry faster.

ALWAYS WASH BRUSHES AND COMBS regularly with hot, soapy water. After cleaning them, place natural bristle brushes face down and leave them to dry naturally. If brushes or combs have broken bristles or teeth, replace them straight away, as prolonged use will tear the hair shaft.

HAIR SOLUTIONS

A balanced diet rich in protein, fresh fruits and vegetables paves the way to general health and great-looking hair.

Hair complaints can result from vitamin and mineral deficiencies. Lack of the vitamin B complex is linked with dandruff and baldness, while the absence of iron can make hair dull and brittle.

Losing 100-200 hairs daily is normal and nothing to be alarmed by.

During pregnancy, hair often looks its best due to hormonal changes. However, about 12 weeks after birth, seemingly excessive hair loss occurs. This is just your hormones rebalancing.

CLEANSING

When faced with hundreds of bottles of shampoos, which one should you choose? Look for a shampoo to suit your needs, taking into consideration the condition and texture of your hair. The safest bet is a pH-balanced shampoo or a mild formulation. These are effective cleansers and won't strip the hair of its essential natural oils.

HAIR SHOULD ONLY BE WASHED on average every third day. Washing too frequently, especially with harsh shampoos, causes the scalp's oil glands to work overtime to compensate for the loss of natural oils. This is the most common cause of greasy hair. Be wary of shampoos that produce a lot of lather, they probably contain high percentages of cheap detergents, which rob the hair of natural oils.

TO INCREASE THE BLOOD FLOW TO YOUR SCALP, bend over a bath or basin when shampooing. Never wash your hair in bath water, as dirty water isn't conducive to clean hair. If you run out of shampoo, don't use dishwashing liquid. It is extremely harsh and will have a drying effect.

CONDITIONING

Just as moisturiser is vital for skin, conditioner is essential for hair. After shampooing, your hair is left with a negative charge and cuticles are dishevelled, making it susceptible to damage. Conditioners contain positively charged agents that bond with the negative charge of cleansed hair. They ensure that the cuticles lie flat and help maintain the hair's overall appearance.

LEAVE-IN CONDITIONERS are an option if you're pushed for time. Designed to help retain moisture in the hair, add shine and reduce static charges, these conditioners are ideal for fine hair (they won't overload it), or to tame flyaway tresses.

CONDITIONERS FOR COLOURED HAIR deposit a protective film around porous, damaged areas of the hair shaft, helping to lock in colour pigments. Special formulations for permed hair give it stability and maintain the curl.

USE A HYDRATING HAIR MASK or treatment once a week to treat very dry hair, or as a post-summer fix. These have far superior conditioning properties than basic conditioners. Protein packs are reconstructive – they put back strength and elasticity into dry, brittle or chemically treated hair, while moisturising treatments make hair softer and more manageable. If you prefer not to leave it to chance, opt for an in-salon service. Professionals use stronger treatments and will prescribe the exact remedy to rectify hair complaints.

HAIR SOLUTIONS

If your favourite shampoo or conditioner comes in a glass bottle and you're worried it will smash in the shower, put rubber bands around the bottle to make it safer and easier to grip.

Don't wash your hair if you're wearing it up. The natural oils in unwashed hair make it easier to style.

Apply conditioner to damp hair for the best results. After shampooing, blot excess water from your hair with a towel.

Avoid using hot oil treatments to hydrate your hair. They are effective but can be difficult to remove. Using excess amounts of shampoo to shift the oil will undo all the good work of the treatment.

Slather on a hair mask or intensive treatment, then wrap your hair in plastic cling wrap and leave it for 10 minutes. The natural heat generated by your body will heighten the power of the conditioning ingredients.

Before swimming, slick wax through your hair. This creates a water-resistant barrier against the elements and helps prevent colour from fading.

Always protect your hair with a styling preparation before exposure to the sun or prior to using heated appliances.

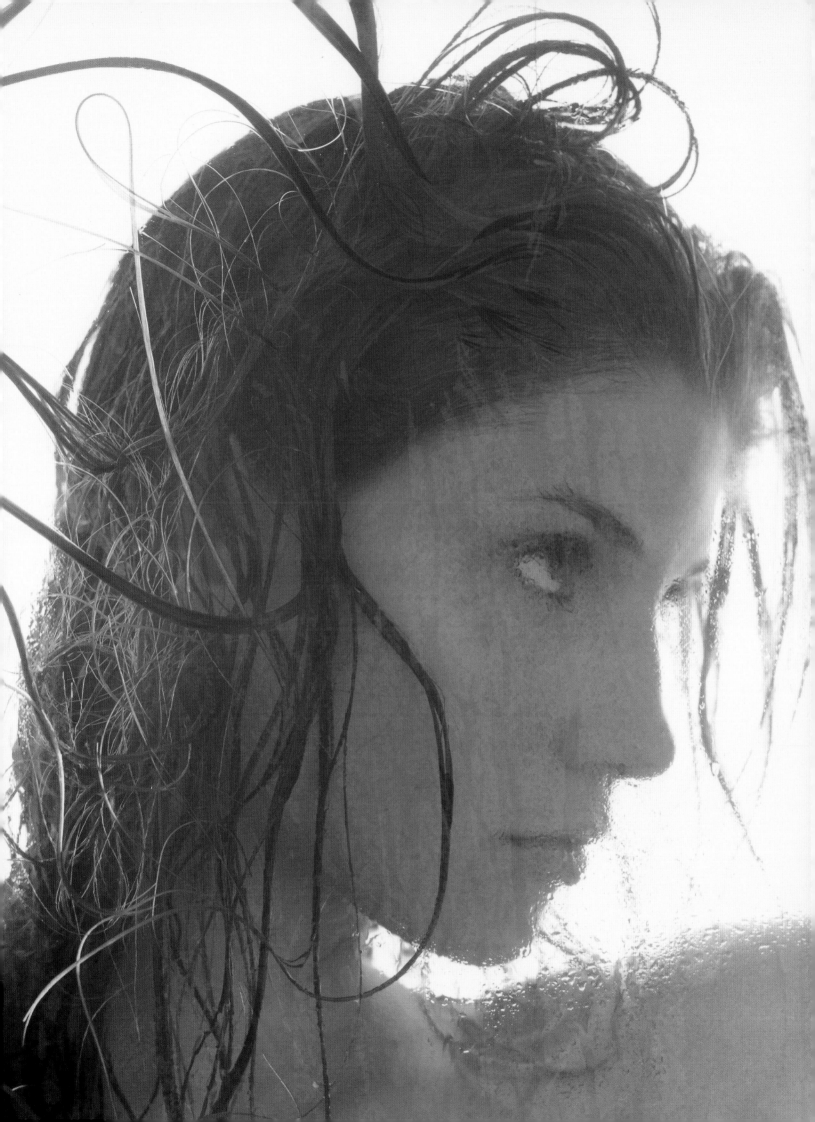

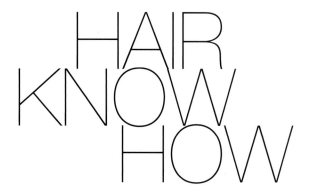

HAIR KNOW HOW

GREASY HAIR

If your hair is greasy, the solution is to add oil. Experts maintain this tricks the scalp into believing that it is actually producing the oil itself, so it will correct the imbalance. Spend a few minutes in a steamy bathroom and then massage 15 drops of jojoba oil (which is similar to the hair's natural oil) into your scalp. Leave it in for 20 minutes and then shampoo. Evaluate your diet – try cutting out dairy produce and fried food.

FRIZZY HAIR

The big frizz is often caused by excess moisture in the atmosphere. To overcome this, use a serum to style your hair. These silicon-based formulas surround the cuticle with a microscopic film that inhibits the absorption of dampness from the surrounding air. Alternatively, use a leave-in conditioner after shampooing. It won't overload the hair and will help it to retain moisture and prevent frizz.

DANDRUFF

Poor diet, sluggish metabolism, hormonal imbalances and infections lead to increased cell renewal on the scalp, commonly known as dandruff. Not to be confused with flaky scalp, dandruff is characterised by scaly particles that have an oily sheen. Washing frequently with a medicated shampoo should stabilise this condition. Alternatively, massage six drops of rosemary oil mixed with 30ml olive oil into your scalp. Leave the oil in overnight and then shampoo it out. If symptoms persist consult a doctor or trichologist.

SPLIT ENDS

Splits ends occur when the cuticle is damaged and the fibres of the cortex unravel as a result of neglect, harsh treatments and chemical processing. No amount of conditioner will repair split ends. The only way to get rid of them is to have them chopped off. To do it yourself, take small sections of hair strands, twist them and carefully use scissors to run up and down the hair shaft, snipping off any stray ends that stick out.

CURLY HAIR

The cuticles of curly hair do not lie flat due to the shape of hair shaft – this often makes curly locks look dull. To overcome this, employ a leave-in conditioner or conditioning spray. This will also enhance curl definition and prevent curly hair from turning into frizz. For a quick fix to revitalise curls, spray your hair with a fine mist of water and scrunch the curls with your hands.

THIN HAIR

Thin hair looks limp and lank when it becomes greasy. Avoid using shampoos enriched with conditioners. Before blow-drying, spritz your hair with a volumising spray that contains polymers – the heat from the dryer swells the polymers, making the hair appear thicker.

LIMP HAIR

To give limp hair more volume, use a can of flat beer as a body-boosting rinse. Dilute one cup of flat beer with three cups of water, pour over the hair, massage thoroughly and then rinse with warm water.

AFRO HAIR

Afro hair is usually dry and brittle, susceptible to damage and difficult to control. Rehydrate with special conditioning preparations formulated for this type of hair and treat your scalp to regular massages to increase the production of the hair's natural hydrating oils.

FLAKY SCALP

A flaky scalp is most commonly spotted when tiny particles of dead skin collect on your shoulders. Often a by-product of stress, lack of sebum, harsh shampoos, vitamin deficiencies and seasonal changes, this condition is easy to rectify. Rebalance a flaky scalp with a moisturising shampoo.

HAIR LOSS

Sudden shock, hormonal changes, stress and illness can all lead to excessive hair loss. Treatments include vitamin and mineral supplements, head massage and relaxation techniques. Consult the experts if you suffer from permanent balding, but be wary of expensive treatments, as they often promise false results.

DRY HAIR

Dry hair is often the result of a dry scalp (where a sufficient supply of sebum is not being produced). To help hydrate dry locks, experts recommend taking vitamin A supplements (take care to follow the recommended amount). Also give your hair and scalp a pre-wash massage with almond or jojoba oil. Leave the oil in for 10 minutes, then apply a mild shampoo and rinse. Brush your hair regularly to stimulate your scalp and distribute existing oils to dry ends.

HAIR SOLUTIONS

If you have greasy hair, colouring is beneficial, as the process changes the porousness of the hair and mops up excess oil.

If you have fine hair, colouring is the ideal option. The hair shaft swells during the chemical processing, making locks appear thicker.

Chemically treated hair shouldn't be washed for at least 48 hours after processing.

After chemical processing, it takes about a month for hair to stabilise, so have a colour or perm well in advance of your holiday.

Coloured hair fades in the sun. Always protect locks from ultraviolet light by wearing a hat or using hair products with sun filters.

To revive your colour use a colour-enhancing shampoo and conditioner once or twice a week. These preparations deposit minuscule colour pigments onto the hair to revitalise and maintain colour.

THE CUTTING EDGE

Investing in a good haircut pays off in the long run, as the overall shape is maintained as your hair grows. There is no set time as to how often hair should be cut, but regular trims every 6–8 weeks will keep it in condition and prevent split ends.

WHEN CONSIDERING A CHANGE OF STYLE, talk to your hairdresser and take into account your hair texture and face shape. There are no strict rules as to what you should and shouldn't have, but bear the following in mind.

ROUND FACES are typified by the equal proportions between the width of the cheekbones and length of the forehead and chin. Balance these proportions with a style that has height at the crown or a short fringe. Steer clear of severe styles that scrape your hair off your face or a mass of curls – they will accentuate the roundness of your face.

SQUARE FACES have a strong jawline and a broad forehead. Opt for longer styles with layers or curls and a side parting. Avoid heavy fringes, centre partings and sharp, jaw-length cuts.

OVAL FACES, characterised by the width of the forehead and cheekbones and a small, pointed chin, are regarded by the experts as the ideal face shape. To balance these features, experiment with a fringe.

LONG FACES, with high foreheads and long chins, require a style that adds width at the sides. Opt for a bob with a fringe, cuts with short layers, or curly styles. Avoid straight, one-length cuts.

PERMING

This delicate operation should be left to the experts. They can analyse the condition of your hair, prescribe the correct perm to suit you and offer a combination of winding techniques to vary the curl definition. You could be faced with numerous disasters if you choose to do your perm at home.

COLOUR

Hair colouring has become so advanced that you can choose to have the most subtle colour enhancement or undergo a drastic transformation. Options are endless, so colour should be an integral part of your haircare regime. For the best results, let the professionals do the work. If you do it yourself, make the task safer by following these guidelines. Rub Vaseline into the skin around your hairline before applying colour. This acts as a protective base to prevent colour from staining the skin. Use an alcohol-based toner and cotton wool to remove any stains on your skin and always wear protective gloves while applying colour. Only leave the product on for the specified time and if the resulting shade is unsightly, seek professional help.

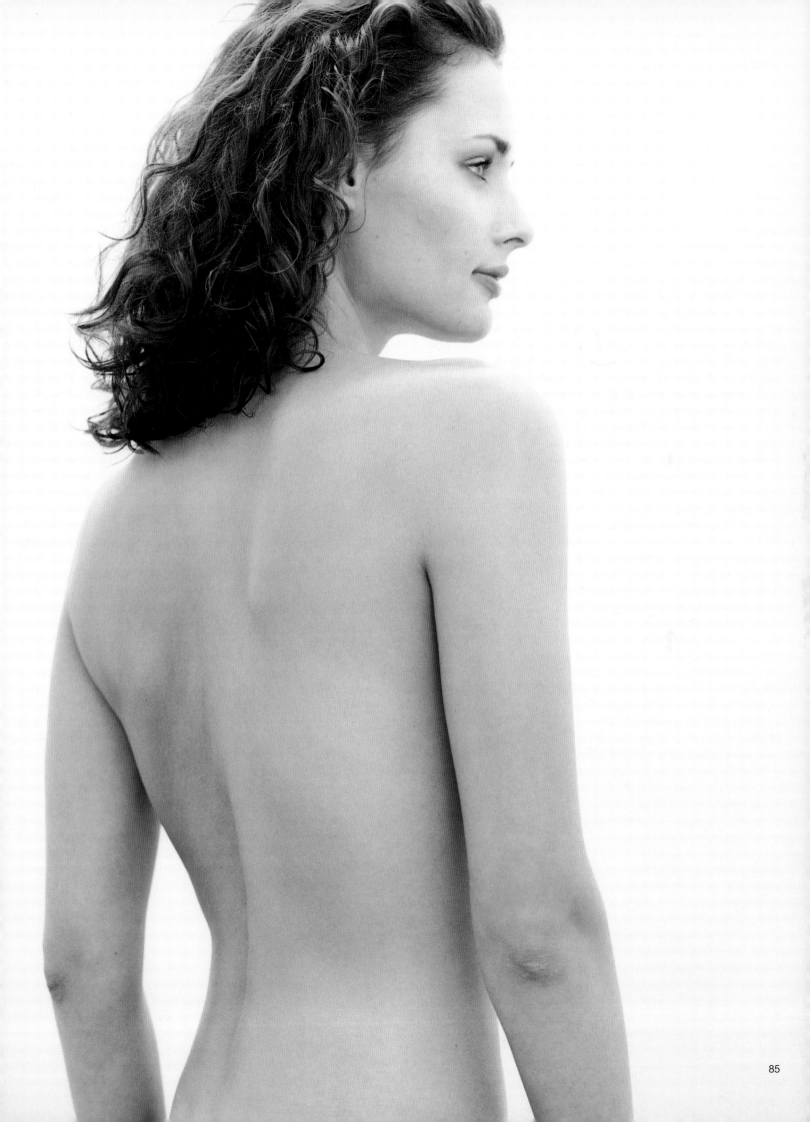

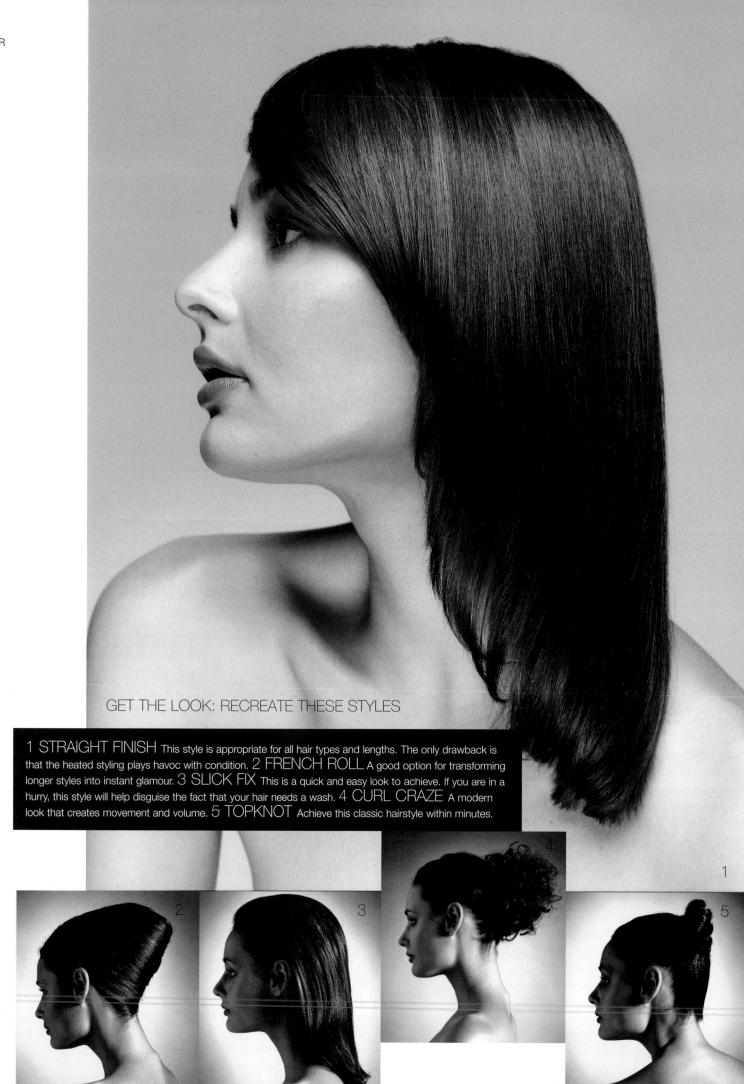

GET THE LOOK: RECREATE THESE STYLES

1 STRAIGHT FINISH This style is appropriate for all hair types and lengths. The only drawback is that the heated styling plays havoc with condition. 2 FRENCH ROLL A good option for transforming longer styles into instant glamour. 3 SLICK FIX This is a quick and easy look to achieve. If you are in a hurry, this style will help disguise the fact that your hair needs a wash. 4 CURL CRAZE A modern look that creates movement and volume. 5 TOPKNOT Achieve this classic hairstyle within minutes.

STYLE FILE

You don't need a hairdresser on hand to master the art of styling. Simply follow these steps to get the look.

STRAIGHT FINISH

Apply mousse to damp hair, comb it through and then partially rough-dry the hair. Next take a 2cm section of hair at the nape of your neck with a comb. Pin the rest of your hair up. Point the airflow of the dryer down the hair shaft, following the brush as you work from the roots to the ends. Ensure each section is dry before taking the next one, working upward. Comb into place and smooth on a pomade or serum to prevent frizz.

FRENCH ROLL

For a modern take on this classic style, comb dry hair and backcomb it at the roots to give extra body if necessary. Then scrape the hair from one side across to the centre of the back of the head. Secure this section of hair with bobby pins, placing them vertically up your head, overlapping or criss-crossing to ensure the hair stays in place. Take the remaining hair and twist it gently. Wrap it over the pins into a roll and tuck the ends under. Secure the hair with pins and spritz it with hair spray.

SLICK FIX

Slicked-back hair is one of the fastest and easiest styles to achieve. Apply gel or pomade to wet or dry hair, comb it through and style with your fingers or a brush. If your hair is long, scrape it back into a ponytail or topknot. If you don't have gel or pomade on hand, use a rich, oil-based moisturiser.

CURL CRAZE

To achieve a modern look, take 2–3cm sections of damp hair. Twist these strands tightly, roll them into a small ball and secure them to your head with a bobby pin, starting at the front of the head and working down to the nape of your neck. Leave the hair to dry naturally or use a blow-dryer to save time. When the hair is completely dry, unravel each section and run your fingers through them. Wear your hair down or in a high ponytail.

TOPKNOT

This is a simple, fast way to put your hair up. Comb your hair into a high ponytail and secure it with an elastic band. (Never use rubber bands as they tear the hair shaft.) Twist the hair around the base of the ponytail to disguise the elastic band and secure it with clips. If you have long hair, twist and literally knot the hair to keep it in place instead of using clips. Experiment by splaying the ends of the hair out of the topknot.

STYLING AGENTS

Hair spray is no longer damaging to the environment or to your hair, providing you select the right brand. Use hair spray to make hair stay in place, tame stray cuticles and help maintain curl definition.

Gel, available in various strengths and formulations ranging from thick gels to pump sprays, can be used on wet hair to sculpt and style; and on dry hair to lift roots, define curls or tame wispy tendrils.

Mousse is a versatile product that can be applied to wet or dry hair to add body and volume. If applied before heat styling, mousse will protect your hair. It is ideal to plump up fine hair and also as a setting agent when creating curls.

Wax and pomades are made from natural waxes, which are softened with other conditioning ingredients. If applied sparingly, they offer instant shine to shorter hair or can be used to tame split ends on longer styles. They are also ideal for slicking hair back as they don't harden like some hair gels. The only drawback with using waxes and pomades is that they can be difficult to remove. To shift these products, apply shampoo to dry hair, add water and then rinse.

Styling spray is an all-in-one product that combines a gel, setting lotion and hair spray. It works well on short styles, for scrunch-drying or to set curls.

Volumising sprays contain special heat-activated ingredients that temporarily plump up fine hair during blow-drying.

Serums, glossers or hair polishes are made from oils or silicon and give hair instant shine, tame frizzy, flyaway locks, smooth cuticles and temporarily seal split ends. To remove these preparations effectively, sprinkle talcum powder into your hair before shampooing to absorb the excess grease. Brush the powder out and then shampoo your hair as normal. A build-up of these products can make the hair look dull and greasy.

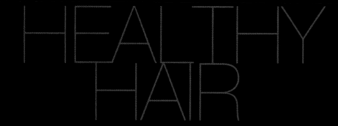

HEALTHY HAIR

FOLLOW THESE STEPS TO ACHIEVE PERFECT CONDITION

BRUSH STROKES

Before shampooing, brush your hair to remove surface dirt and any tangles. Forget the myth that brushing 100 strokes daily is beneficial. Over-vigorous brushing can tear and generally weaken the hair shaft.

CLEANSE EASE

Take short cuts to remove any build-up of styling products in your hair. Massage shampoo into dry hair and rinse it out with warm water. This will be sufficient to remove impurities and your hair shouldn't need another wash.

SCALP TREAT

Massage your scalp in the shower to boost circulation, improve hair health and reduce stress. Knead your scalp gently using the pads of your fingers. Start at the front of your head and work down to the nape of your neck.

MOIST HAIR

Only apply conditioner to the ends and mid-lengths of your hair, (the hair near your scalp should have enough natural hydrating oils). Applying conditioner near the roots will make your hair feel greasy shortly after washing.

FINAL RINSE

Boost hair shine and remove tangles by using vinegar as a rinse after shampooing. Dilute one tablespoon of vinegar in 600ml tepid water and pour it over your hair. Comb it through and then rinse it out with warm water.

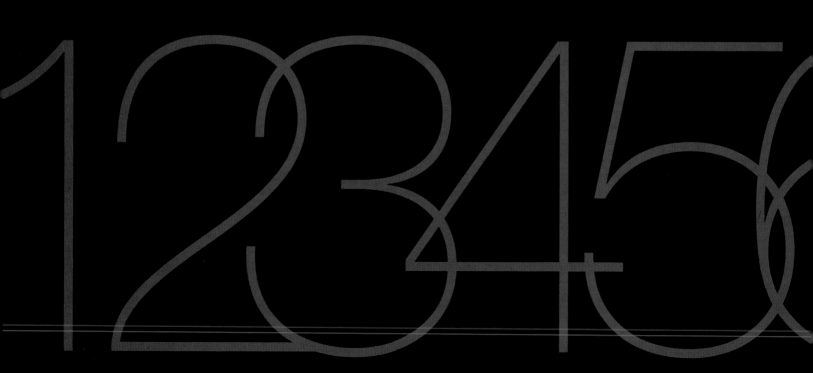

WATER WORKS

Hot water causes the cuticles to swell, creating an uneven surface and making locks appear dull. Use cold water to rinse your hair. The coldness of the water will close the cuticles, ensuring all-over hair shine.

SQUEEZE EASE

Never towel dry your hair, as it robs the locks of moisture and destroys elasticity. Squeeze excess water from the hair using your fingertips and then blot the hair with a towel. This helps to retain vital moisture.

TANGLE FREE

Never brush wet hair. It is swollen to twice its normal size and is susceptible to damage. Use a wide-tooth comb and work through wet hair in sections, starting with the ends. Comb your hair until it is completely tangle-free.

STYLING SENSE

Leave your tresses to dry naturally, as heated styling appliances damage the hair shaft. Twist long hair into a topknot and leave it to set as the hair dries. Apply a small amount of gel to short hair and comb it through.

CUTICLE TAMER

Once your hair is dry, spray a fine mist of hair spray onto a comb and run it through the hair. This will tame any stray cuticles or flyaway ends and give the hair a neat, polished finish, ensuring long-lasting perfection for your hairstyle.

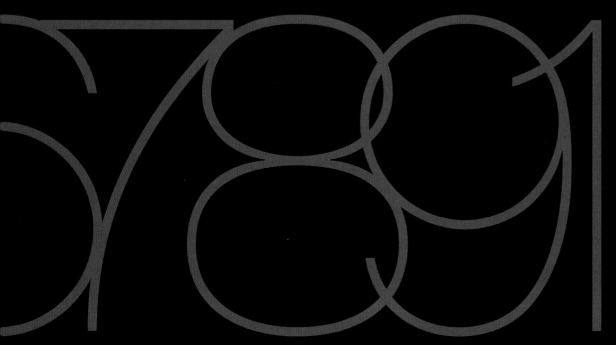
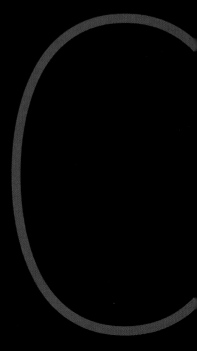

PROBLEM

Can you temporarily tame split ends?

For a quick fix to disguise unsightly ends, seal them with a slick of Vaseline.

Shortly after you've shampooed your hair, does it look greasy?

Check the water temperature. Avoid rinsing your hair with hot water because this disrupts the balance of the scalp by increasing oil production.

Can you take short cuts to curling your hair?

Spray your hair with setting lotion and put rollers in before bathing or showering (wear a shower cap). The steam from the water will help set the curls. Only remove the rollers when your hair is completely dry.

How can you control static, flyaway hair?

An anti-static clothes spray tames flyaway hair just as well as it works on clothes. Rather than applying it directly to your hair, spray some onto a hair brush and then brush it through.

Will regular trims make your hair grow faster?

Contrary to popular belief, having regular cuts will not make your hair grow more quickly. Hair grows from inside the scalp at a rate of about one centimetre per month.

Do you always wake up with bed-head hair?

This is where a satin pillowcase is especially useful: it helps to keep hair in place. Hair moves smoothly over satin, whereas cotton causes friction and frizz.

Does your hair look dull and lifeless?

Try changing your shampoo and conditioner. Prolonged use of the same products can cause a residue build-up on the hair shaft.

Does your hair have an unsightly green tinge after swimming?

Chlorinated water has a tendency to turn natural and not-so-natural blonde hair an unsightly shade of green. To rectify discolouration, use tomato juice as a colour-correcting rinse.

What is the best way to remove sand, salt and impurities from your hair?

To help shift impurities, pour soda water over your hair before shampooing.

Should you use lemon juice to lighten your hair while in the sun?

Lemon juice is a perfect agent for sun-kissed brightening, but it plays havoc with hair condition. To counteract the drying effects of the lemon juice, mix it with conditioner before smoothing it on.

SOLUTION

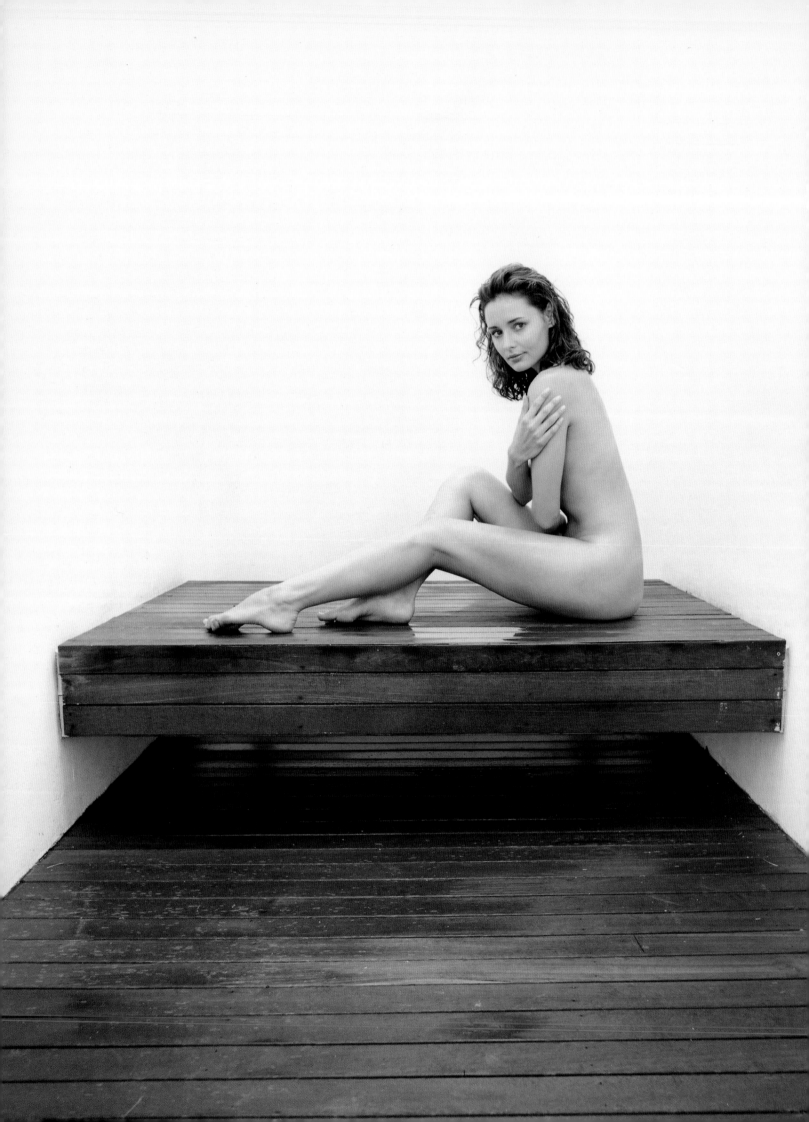

BODY

Body

MAINTENANCE SHOULD BE AN INTEGRAL PART OF ANY BEAUTY REGIME. ENHANCING THE APPEARANCE OF YOUR BODY WILL IMPROVE YOUR SELF-IMAGE AND SELF-ESTEEM.

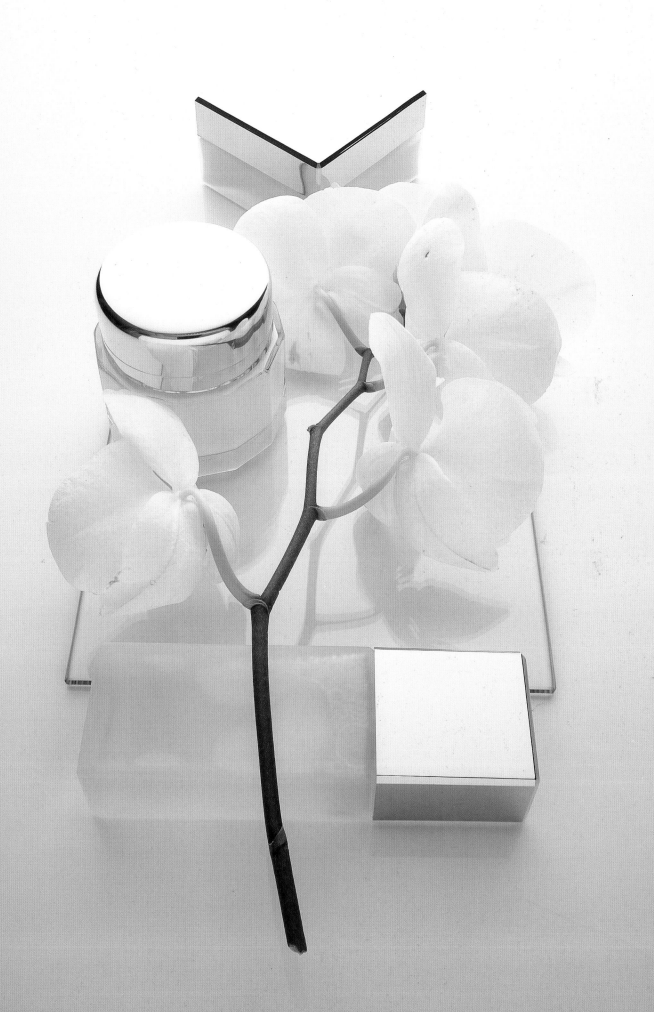

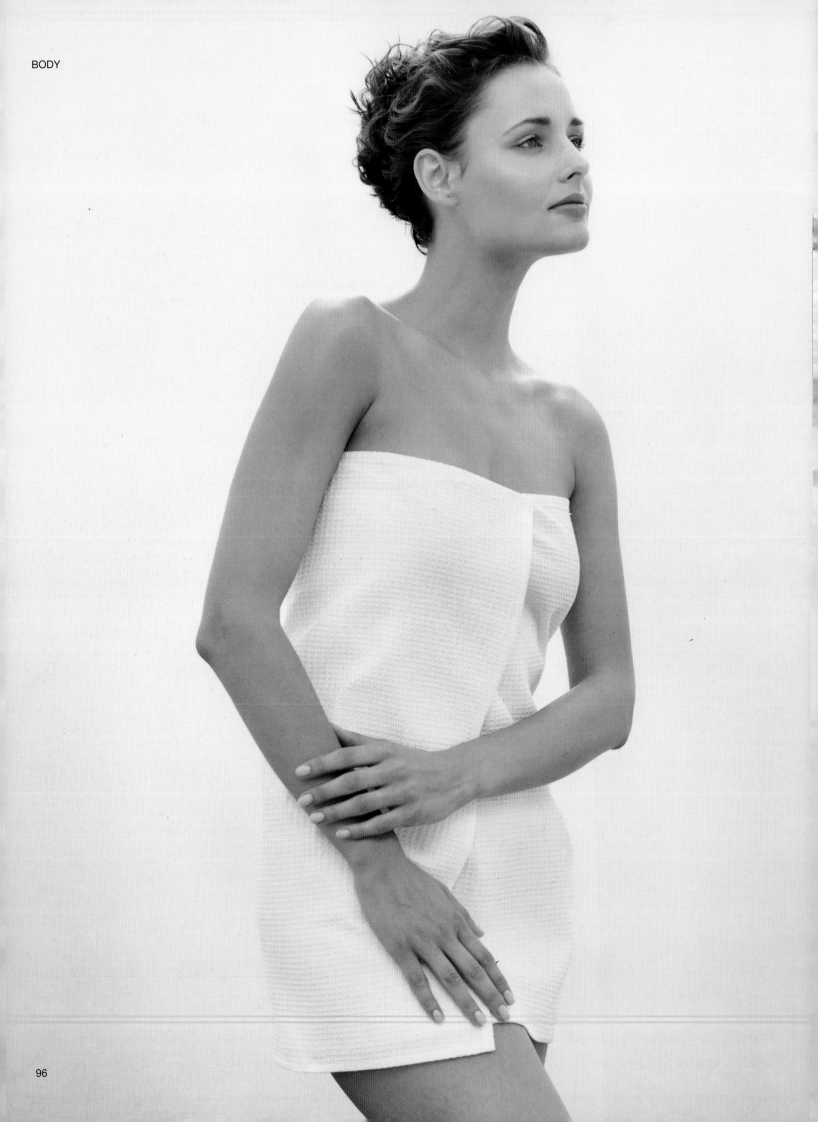

BODY MAINTENANCE

Tending to your body's outer beauty needs is just as important as looking after your face. If you are scrupulous about applying facial moisturiser, why would you neglect hydrating your body? If you look after the delicate skin around your eyes, why would you overlook your décolleté? Apart from making you look good and feel good, many body treatments are more than skin-deep. They can shift unwanted toxins and boost circulation to improve your general health. Pampering your body also provides the perfect opportunity to switch off, relax and completely unwind.

EXFOLIATION

On average your skin naturally renews itself every 28 days, but this process slows down as you age. Dead cells build up, making your skin look dull and feel rough. Regular exfoliation gives your skin a polished finish and increases circulation. Use a loofah, body mitt or scrub to massage damp skin, working over your body in small, circular motions. Pay attention to areas that are prone to dryness, such as your knees, elbows and feet. For the best results, aim to exfoliate your skin once or twice a week.

BODY BRUSHING

Dry skin brushing is a more intense form of exfoliation. While whisking away dead cells, the brush strokes also stimulate lymphatic drainage and eliminate as much as one third of your body's wastes. Dry skin brushing also offers your body the same stimulation as a good massage or 20 minutes' exercise (although it should not replace physical activity). Before showering, use a soft-bristled brush and work over your body (but not your face) using long, sweeping movements. Start at the soles of your feet and work up your legs. Then work on your arms and torso, brushing up towards your heart. Work over your abdomen in clockwise strokes. Start with gentle pressure and as your skin becomes used to the sensation, increase the pressure. When you finish brushing, take a warm shower and then smooth moisturiser all over your body. As a result of the body's purification process, you may find that the odd pimple appears on your skin after brushing.

BODY SOLUTIONS

Create a body scrub by mixing a handful of oatmeal and bran with a little rose water. Massage this mixture into damp skin and then rinse it off.

If you use a body brush, wash it regularly in warm, soapy water to remove impurities and dead skin cells.

If you have sensitive skin, rub a towel over your body instead of a body brush. This will be more gentle on delicate skin.

Don't exfoliate or brush areas of skin prone to disorders such as psoriasis, eczema, varicose veins or any patches of broken skin. Instead, work around them.

If you brush your skin daily, take a week's break every month. Otherwise your body becomes used to the treatment, making it less effective.

Care for neglected skin with a double-strength exfoliating treat. First massage a scrub into damp skin, then work over your body with a mitt or loofah while you are in the shower.

BATHING

Soaking in a bathtub can be a therapeutic experience for both mind and body. Warm water dissipates aches and pains and eases tension, so the temperature of the water should be approximately 35°C. If it is any hotter, your pulse rate will increase, making you feel drained and weak after bathing.

AROMATHERAPY OILS added to the bath can aid everything from skin complaints to muscle fatigue, depending on your needs (see page 182). Always add oil to the bath after the water has run and then stir the water to disperse the droplets.

A SALT BATH is reputed to enhance a body-cleansing regime. Before going to bed, run a warm bath and add 250g Epsom salts and 250g sea salt. Relax for 10–15 minutes, topping up the warm water when necessary. Do not use soap as this interferes with the activity of the salts. Afterwards, pat your skin dry and get into a pre-heated bed. Expect to sweat profusely and sleep deeply – this is all part of the detoxification process. Ensure that you have a glass of water at hand to help replenish lost liquid. Have this type of treatment once a month.

HYDRATION

Just as your face requires moisturiser, so does your body. After showering or bathing, always slather on a hydrating preparation while the skin is slightly damp. If you're pushed for time, use a body spray for hydration. They are easy to apply and quickly absorbed by the skin. For an indulgent experience, use a scented body lotion that matches your existing fragrance.

GIVE YOURSELF A QUICK MASSAGE while applying moisturiser if you have the time. This is a good opportunity to boost circulation, tackle cellulite, reduce water retention and alleviate stress all at once. Use the following basic massage movements to work on the problem zones of your body: start and end a massage with light, gentle strokes known as *effleurage*, which relax and warm the muscles. Then work on problem areas with *petrissage*, deep rhythmic, kneading movements. Using your fingertips and palms, these stimulating movements help to disperse toxin build-up in the skin cells. Follow with *tapotement*, invigorating slapping and cupping movements that improve overall muscle tone. (For self-massage, see page 178.)

BODY SOLUTIONS

If you have dry skin, add two tablespoons of sweet almond oil to your bath, as well as your choice of essential oil.

If you have sunburnt skin, have a cool bath laced with eight drops of camomile oil and eight tablespoons of cider vinegar to soothe your skin. Never apply pure essential oils to burnt skin.

If you have a headache, relax in a warm bath and put a steaming hot towel around your neck and shoulders to ease the pain.

Customise body products by mixing fragrance-free moisturiser with a few drops of your favourite perfume.

Enrich moisturiser by mixing it with a capsule of vitamin E oil.

If you run out of moisturiser use wheatgerm oil instead. It's similar in structure to the skin's natural lubricant, sebum, and is enriched with vitamins A, B, C and E, which condition your skin.

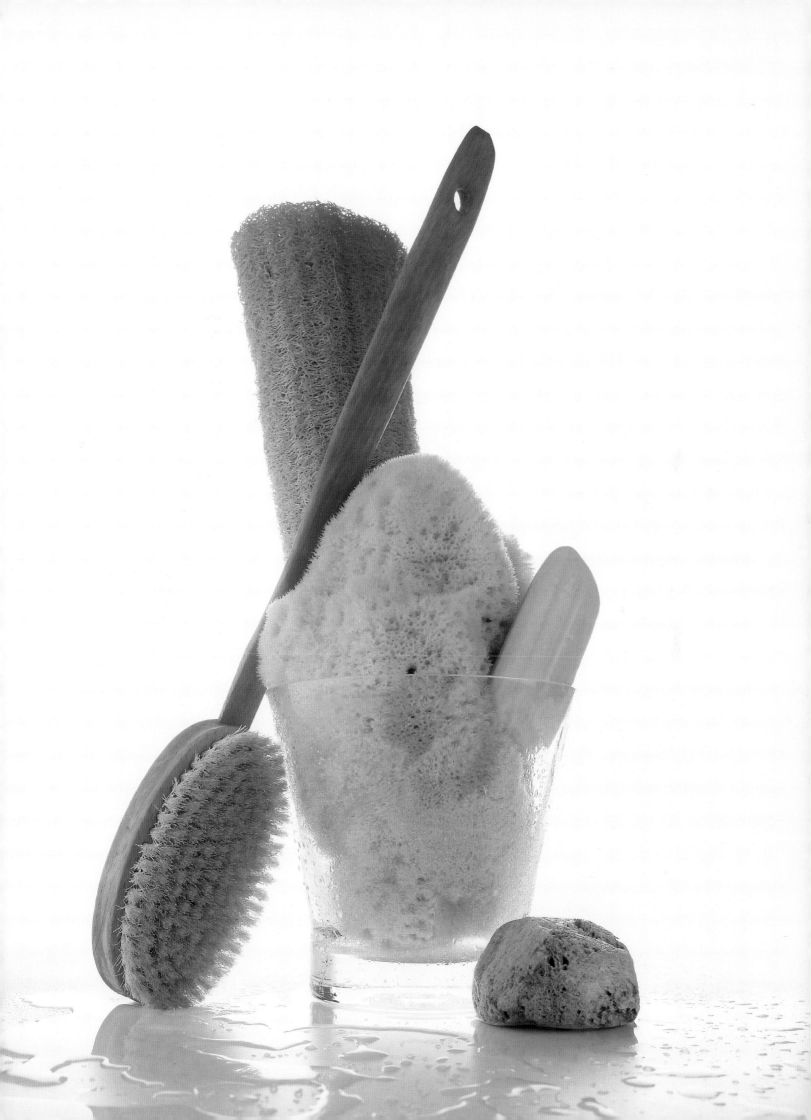

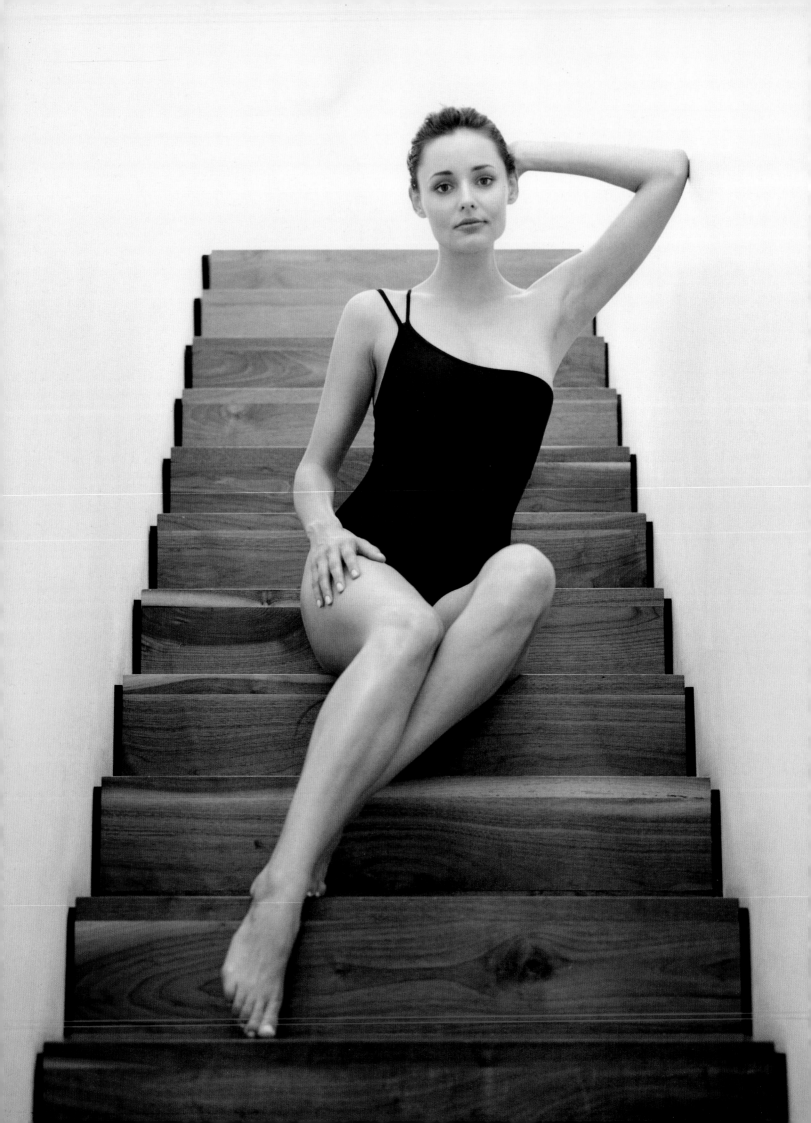

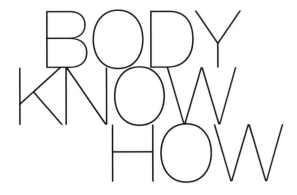

BODY KNOW HOW

Improve the appearance of your body by tackling problems with the latest beautifying treatments and take preventative steps to help maintain your overall body condition.

STRETCH MARKS

Stretch marks usually occur on the breasts and abdomen due to weight increase, during pregnancy or as a result of vitamin deficiencies. There is apparently no cure for stretch marks, but to lessen their appearance ensure that you have an adequate intake of zinc, silica and vitamin B6 in your diet and apply pure vitamin E oil to your skin. To temporarily disguise any marks, use a waterproof make-up base.

BODY ODOUR

On average you lose one litre of water through perspiration each day. Sweating is your body's temperature control and waste disposal mechanism. Perspiration is actually odourless when it leaves your body – it only begins to smell when it comes into contact with bacteria, usually after about six hours. Antiperspirants block the pores to prevent sweating, which is not ideal as it can lead to toxin build-up. Deodorants are safer to use as they merely disguise the smell.

HAIR REMOVAL

Removing excess body hair can be tedious. Shaving is the quickest and easiest way to achieve smooth, hair-free legs and underarms. Instead of using shaving gels or creams, simply use hair conditioner – it does the job and helps condition your skin at the same time. Waxing is the best method of hair removal as regrowth can take up to six weeks to appear. If you can't stand the pain of waxing or want a permanent solution, there are treatments available that use lasers to zap hairs at the roots. After a course of these treatments, excess hair should have disappeared but it's a costly procedure.

VARICOSE VEINS

Swollen and knotted superficial veins can be hereditary, or they can develop in association with pregnancy, obesity, vitamin deficiencies or as a result of standing for prolonged periods. To prevent varicose veins, eat fibre-rich foods and drink at least two litres of water daily. Avoid crossing your legs and standing for long periods and put your feet up regularly. Varicose veins can be removed with sclerotherapy.

POSTURE

Good posture goes hand-in-hand with a better self-image. If you spend hours slaving over a computer, bending over or carrying heavy loads, it's likely that your posture is out of balance, which can affect the proper functioning of the rest of your organs. Specific therapies performed under guidance focus on realigning the body to maintain optimum health.

Pilates promotes better body awareness through exercises that readdress muscle tone and balance. It works by stimulating the muscles opposite to those that are overworked. To accompany each movement, rhythmic breathing helps to release tension and rids the body of waste products.

Rolfing employs deep, sometimes painful, massage movements that manipulate the muscles' connective tissue to restore harmony to every part of the body.

The Alexander Technique addresses the mind–body link and looks at how stress and emotions affect the body's alignment. Much emphasis is placed on the region at the base of the neck, where nerve fibres transmit information about the state of the body's muscles and joints to the brain. When the muscles in this area become tense, the body falls out of balance. The Alexander Technique helps to control this imbalance.

CELLULITE

There is no miracle cure (apart from liposuction) to eradicate orange-peel thighs. Slathering on cream is not going to shift stubborn patches of cellulite. However, with an effective beauty regime, a healthy, nutritionally balanced diet and regular exercise, you can expect to see an improvement. Steer clear of alcohol, sugar, butter and animal fats, dairy produce and excess amounts of salt.

THREAD VEINS

Thread veins can be hereditary, or the result of sun damage, excess weight loss or pregnancy. If you suffer from networks of surface veins, avoid saunas and steer clear of hot water as these aggravate the condition. A short course of sclerotherapy will remove these veins. A fine needle is injected into the vein to expel the blood, causing the walls of the vein to stick together. This stops the blood from flowing back in. Sclerotherapy is relatively painless and the only after-effect is a little bruising which lasts for several days. Thread veins can also be removed with laser treatments.

TARGET ZONES

BREASTS & DÉCOLLETÉ

Often neglected, the delicate skin of the bust and décolleté is susceptible to signs of ageing. A five-minute daily massage with a bust-care preparation will improve your skin's texture and help postpone sagging. To massage, put one hand behind your head and using the other hand, work around the breasts in a figure of eight. Repeat using the other hand.

VISUALLY AND MANUALLY EXAMINE YOUR BREASTS once a month, preferably the day after your period ends. Watch for variations in nipple size, dimpling of the skin and any colour changes. Then either stand or lie down and use the pads of your fingers to examine each breast, pressing firmly and working in small, circular motions. Start at the outside of the breast, working inwards in a spiral towards the nipple. Then work up to the décolleté and under the armpit. If you locate any suspicious lumps, consult a doctor for a thorough examination. The majority of breast lumps are benign.

UPPER BODY

Because of the amount of oil-producing glands on the back and shoulders, blemishes can be a common occurrence. Use a body brush or loofah to exfoliate this area, wash it with a medicated cleansing bar and then zap blemishes by dabbing on lavender oil. For serious conditions, see a doctor.

THE UPPER BODY, ESPECIALLY THE ARMS, is a common site for malignant moles. Keep a check on any freckles and moles on your torso and the rest of your body. If you notice any changes, always have them checked by the experts.

HIPS & THIGHS

To keep your hips and thighs in shape, blitz them with a high-powered jet of water from the shower head. To break down cellulite and shift unwanted toxins, alternate the water temperature from warm to cold. Mountain biking, step aerobics and running will also help tone this region of your body.

ASSESS YOUR DIET. It's true that what passes through the lips ends up on the hips and thighs. Research shows that specific foods are linked with cellulite. Avoid sugars and starches, choose chicken and fish instead of red meat, steer clear of animal fats such as butter and limit your consumption of salt and spices. Increase your intake of fresh fruits and vegetables.

LEG CARE

Beautiful legs thrive on two simple strategies: exfoliating and moisturising. Your legs have fewer sebaceous glands than the rest of your body, so they are prone to dryness, especially on the shins. Keep moisture levels on your legs topped up and exfoliate regularly.

IF YOU HAVE TO STAND FOR LONG PERIODS, rock to and fro on the balls of your feet to boost circulation and rotate each ankle to help the calf muscles pump blood back up your legs. If you have to sit down for hours, the flow of blood to the legs slows down, causing swollen feet and calves. To avoid this, get up regularly and walk around.

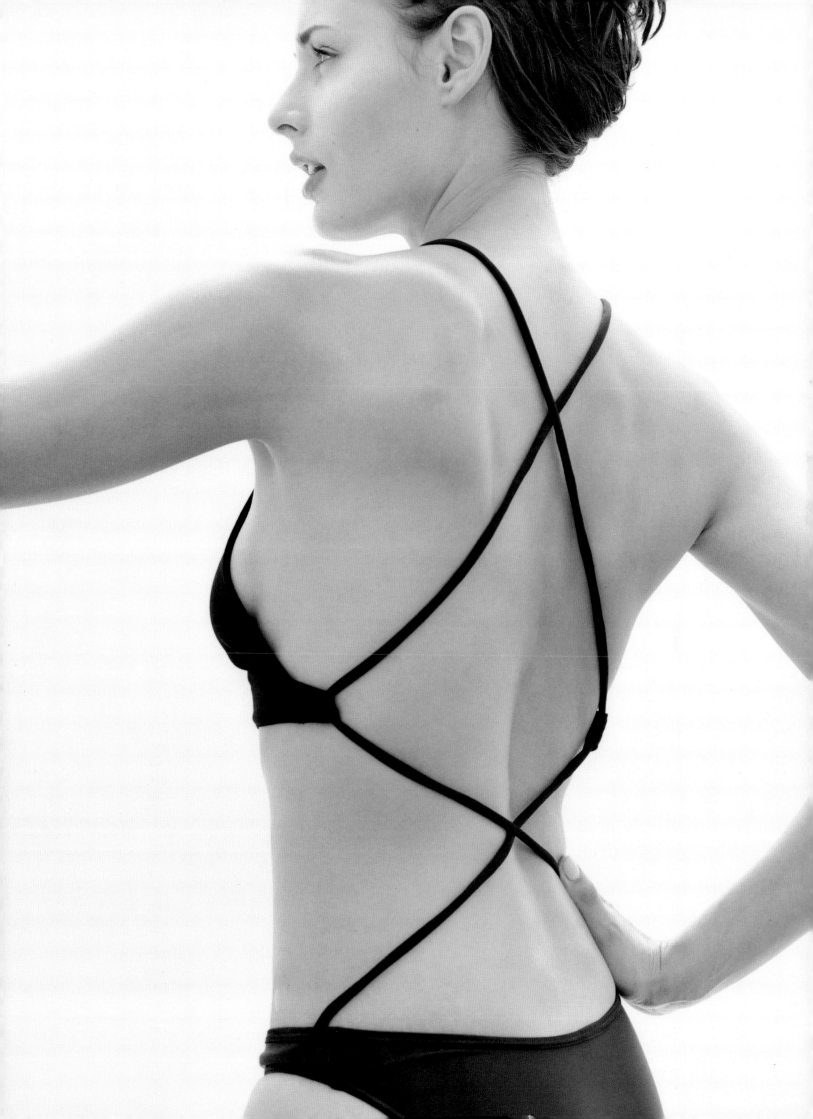

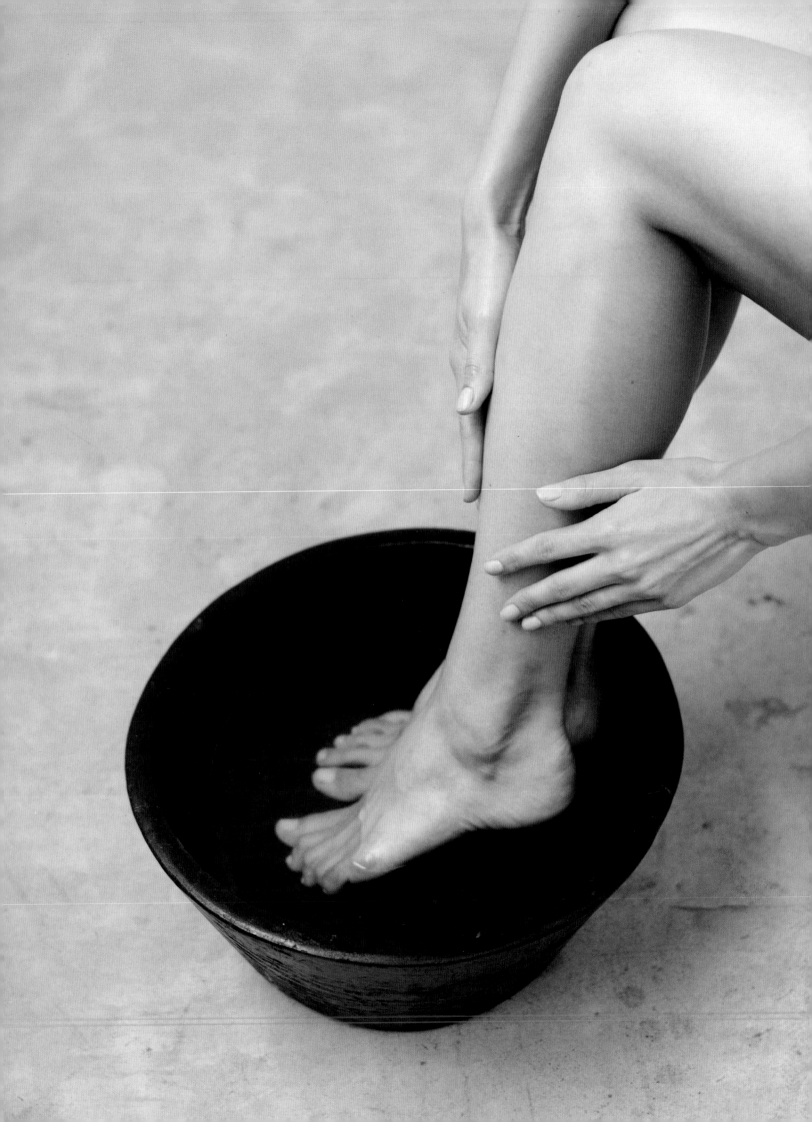

HANDS

Pay special attention to your hands when tending to your beauty needs. Exfoliate them regularly to remove dry skin and slather on hand cream. Use a preparation containing sunscreen whilst outdoors.

FINGER EXERCISES can help prevent Occupational Overuse Syndrome (OOS), formerly known as Repetitive Strain Injury (RSI). This syndrome occurs from constant, repetitive actions, such as typing. Exercise your fingers by clenching them into a ball, then slowly release them and stretch the fingers out. Rotate your wrists in circular motions.

TREAT YOURSELF TO A MANICURE each week. When shaping your nails, file in one direction only to prevent causing damage to the nail plate. Leaving old nail polish on while filing your nails will help protect them.

REMOVE OLD NAIL POLISH using an acetone formula. Press a cotton wool pad soaked in nail polish remover onto the nail plate for a few seconds, allowing the remover to soak through the polish. It can then be removed easily in one wipe.

TO TREAT CUTICLES, soak your fingers in warm water mixed with one tablespoon of olive oil for 10 minutes. Then use an orange stick or cotton bud to push the cuticles back gently. Never trim them with cuticle clippers. Wash your hands with warm water (not soap), then dry them thoroughly with a tissue. This removes any residue in preparation for polish application.

TO APPLY NAIL POLISH, paint one stripe down the centre of the nail from the base to the nail tip, then paint one brush stroke on either side, avoiding the nail edges. This elongates the nail and makes your fingers look slender. For the best results, apply two coats of polish. If you're wearing coloured varnish, always use a base coat to prevent staining the nail plate.

FEET

Care for your feet by exfoliating them regularly. After relaxing in a bath for 10 minutes, get to work on your soles with a pumice stone. Gently exfoliate, working in small, circular motions to remove stubborn patches of dry skin.

GIVE YOURSELF A REGULAR PEDICURE. Soak your feet in a bowl of warm water laced with a few drops of lavender or almond oil. Exfoliate your feet and gently scrub the cuticles with a nail brush. Cut your toenails straight across and smooth the edges with the coarse side of an emery board. Paint your nails with a polish of your choice.

BODY SOLUTIONS

Nail polish can take over eight hours to dry until it's dent-proof. Paint your nails before going to bed to allow maximum drying time.

Protect your hands by wearing cotton-lined gloves when gardening or doing household chores and wear rubber gloves when washing up.

To strengthen your nails, always wear a coat of clear polish.

French-manicure your nails by painting the tip of each nail with white polish. Leave them to dry and then apply another coat to the nail tip. Finish with a layer of clear polish over the entire nail.

For odour-free feet, wipe your soles with surgical spirit twice a day.

A foot massage can be a tonic for your entire body. Apply moisturiser or body oil and knead the sole of each foot. Then work over the top of the foot and up the leg with long sweeping motions.

To relieve aching feet, rub your soles with cider vinegar or lemon juice.

Ill-fitting shoes are best avoided as they can cause problems later in life.

For a skin-softening treat, smooth a thin film of Vaseline onto your feet and wear a pair of cotton socks to bed. The heat generated will intensify the skin-softening properties of the Vaseline.

BODY WORK

FOLLOW THESE STEPS TO ACHIEVE TOP-TO-TOE BEAUTY

BRONZE LIMBS

Lightly tanned flesh can enhance your overall look, especially if it's toned and supple.
To give your legs a flattering finish, apply self-tan. It can create the illusion that legs are longer and leaner than they really are.

SUSTAIN WEIGHT

Avoid faddish diets and eat sensibly, as a loss or increase of 2kgs can stretch your skin. Maintain skin suppleness and help tone down stretch marks by smoothing on lotions containing vitamin E or cocoa butter.

BODY REALIGN

Take note of your posture: slouching makes you look shorter and standing straight makes your stomach look flatter. Bad body alignment will also affect the proper functioning of your organs.

PERFECT SIZING

If your bra doesn't fit properly, it can restrict circulation, give limited support and leave you with unsightly looking bulges. Have your bust measured professionally and invest in a bra that fits properly and offers the correct support.

SLEEP TIGHT

Get a sufficient amount of sleep as the body regenerates itself during the night. Ensure a peaceful night's sleep by massaging the soles of your feet with sesame seed or coconut oil before going to bed.

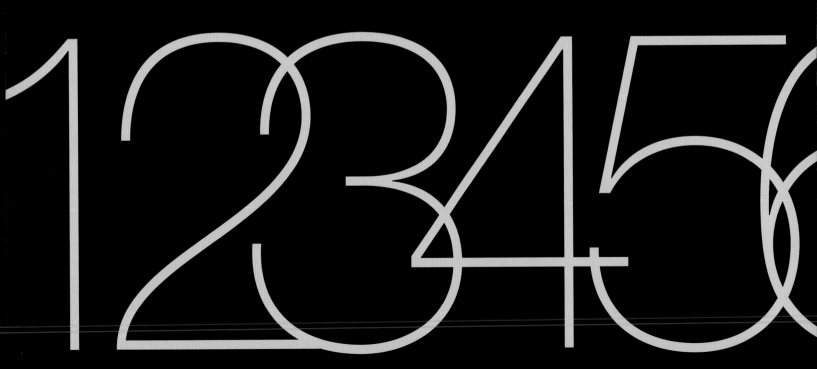

PHYSICAL NOTIONS

Exercise regularly. Aim to incorporate at least 30 minutes of aerobic activity into your routine three times each week and also do muscle toning work such as yoga. This combination of activity improves your body and overall health.

WATER WORKS

Maintain healthy skin and regulate the functioning of your body's organs by drinking one to one and a half litres of water a day. On average, 10 cups of water a day are lost via evaporation, sweating and breathing.

VARYING HEIGHTS

Vary the height of heels you wear to avoid bad circulation, backache, muscle fatigue and poor posture. To take the strain off your feet, use cushioned insoles or make an effort to walk around without wearing shoes.

GOLDEN RULES

If you use fake tan, apply it carefully and ensure that you blend it thoroughly. A bronzed complexion and white earlobes will give the game away, and tanned legs and pale arms will leave you looking like a two-tone beauty.

FIRMING TREAT

Keep your bust in trim with simple wide-arm push-ups, breast stroke or training with light weights to strengthen the underlying muscles of your breasts. Good posture also plays a vital role in preventing the big sag.

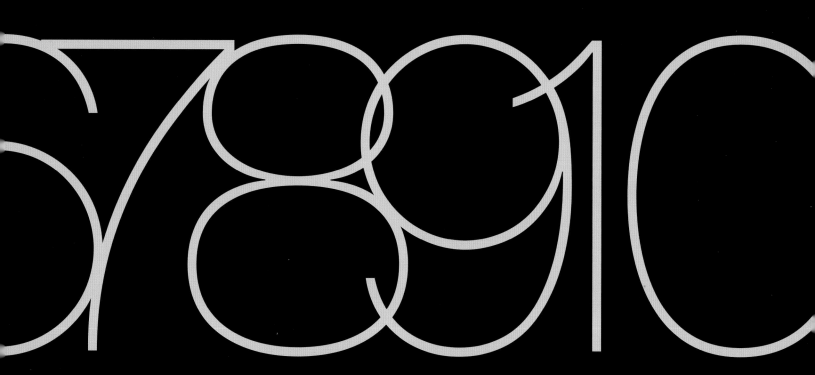

PROBLEM

What hydrates your skin if you run out of moisturiser?
Employ hair conditioner to do the job – the creamy consistency is a great substitute.

How can you prevent ingrown hairs?
Minimise ingrown hairs by using the hot wax rather than strip wax method of hair removal. Use a body scrub three times a week between waxes and always moisturise skin after bathing.

Do you need to splash out on fancy exfoliating products?
A handful of sea salt massaged into damp skin will work just as effectively as expensive scrubs.

Is wallowing in the bath **good for you?**
Limit your time in the tub to a maximum of 20 minutes as prolonged soaking dries the skin out. Make sure the water temperature is less than 35°C.

When should you apply self-tanning products?
Apply self-tanning preparations before going to bed so the colour can develop as you sleep. Avoid application straight after waxing or shaving your legs as the result will be uneven.

How can you give bare legs a flattering finish?

Blend moisturiser with a small amount of foundation and smooth the mixture onto your skin.

How can you relieve swollen ankles?

To reduce swelling, drink spring water, but steer clear of tap or mineral water. These contain sodium, a mineral that increases water retention.

Is there a solution to disguise streaky self-tan lines?

Smooth whitening toothpaste onto streaky marks and leave for several minutes to lighten discolouration. Rinse off with warm water.

Can you temporarily create a bigger cleavage?

To accentuate a cleavage, make-up artists recommend using a bronze lipstick and drawing a line down between the breasts, then blending it into the skin with the fingertips.

How can you ease shaving rash?

Use a cotton wool pad douched with camomile lotion to soothe irritation and reduce redness.

SOLUTION

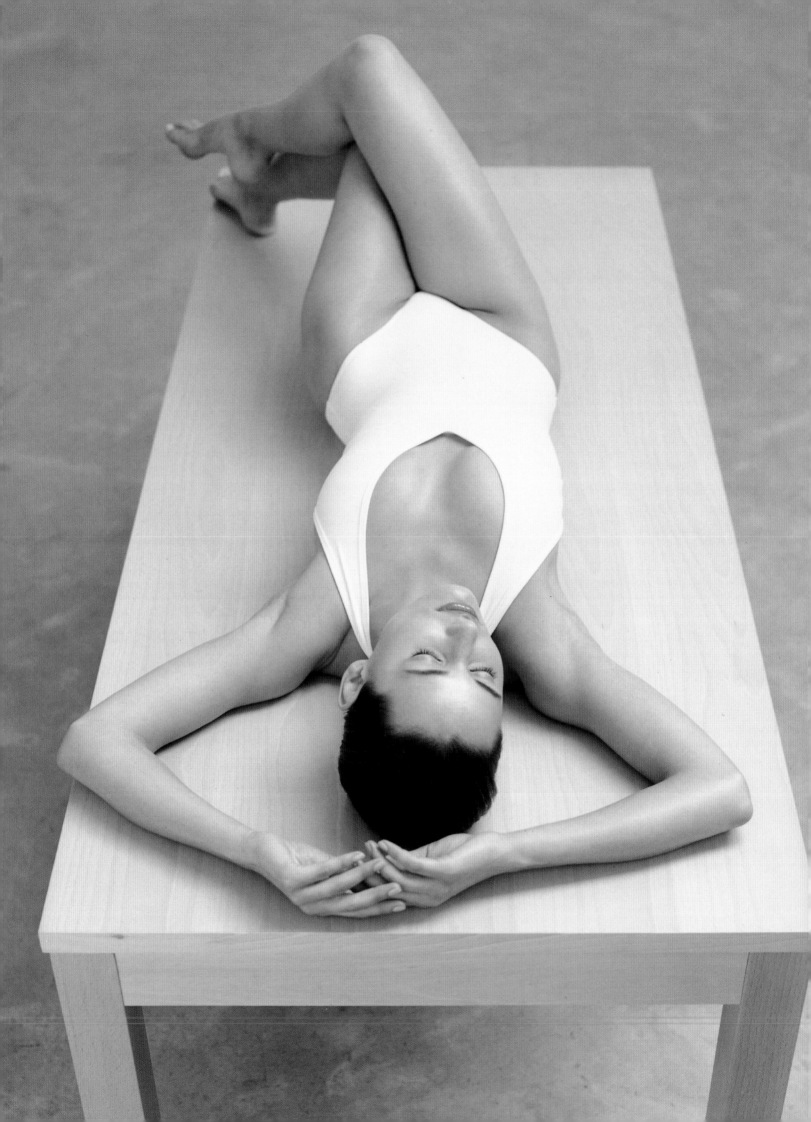

HOME SPA

Health

SPAS OFFER RELAXATION AND PROMOTE WELL-BEING. INTRODUCE THE SPA PHILOSOPHY INTO YOUR OWN HOME AND REAP THE THERAPEUTIC BENEFITS FOR YOUR MIND, BODY AND SPIRIT.

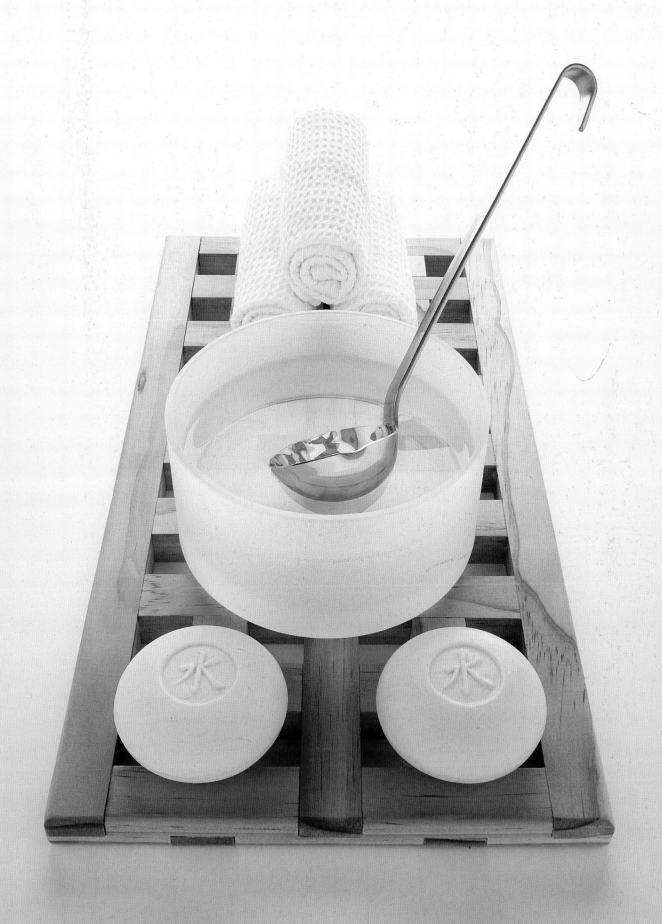

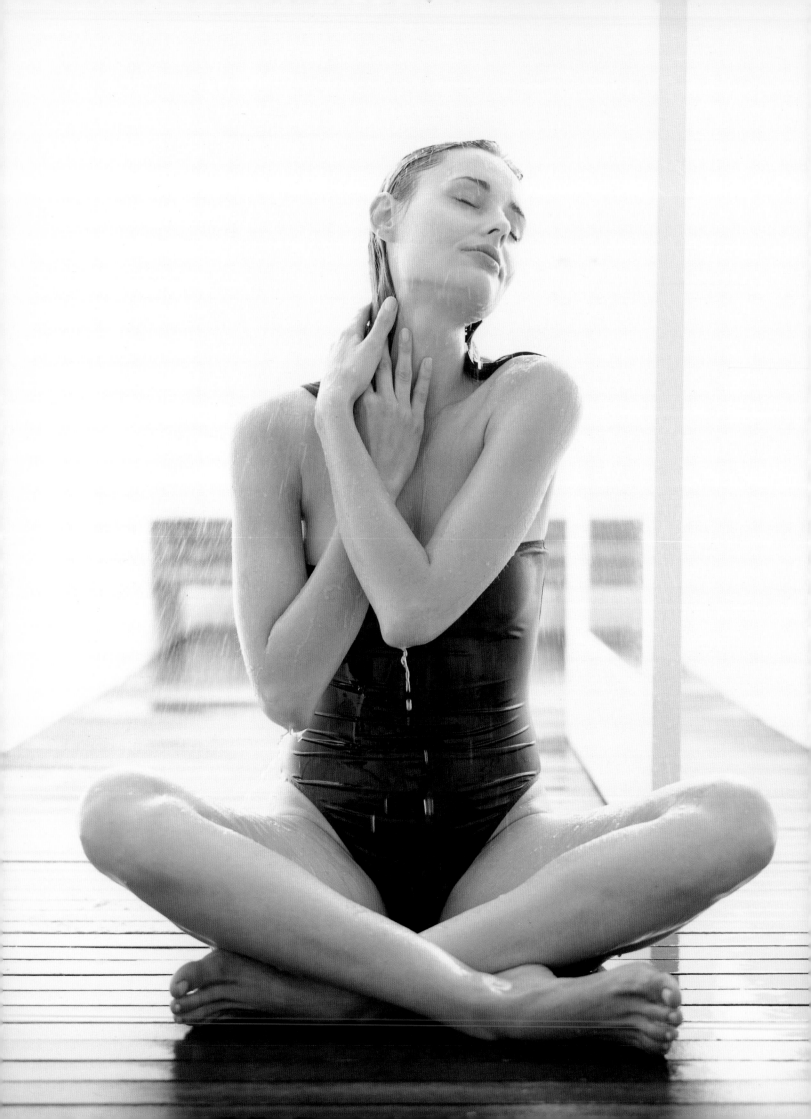

HEALTH SPAS

Health spas have been around for centuries. (The word 'spa' originates from the Belgian town of Spa, which was a fashionable mineral spring resort in the 18th century.) Spas differ in their approach to well-being and specialise in various beautifying treatments, but they all aim to offer one thing: a tonic for the stresses and strains of modern living. Nutritious foods, relaxation, pampering treats, soul-enhancing therapies and exercise are all part of spa life. You can now reap these benefits in the comfort of your own home with DIY treatments and nutritious, spa-inspired meals.

SPA TREATS

Most spa treatments take their cue from nature and employ the natural benefits of the sea and mineral springs.

THALASSOTHERAPY (from the Greek *thalassa*, meaning sea), incorporates sea water in a variety of different treatments. Sea water is a rich source of minerals (such as iron and zinc), trace elements and marine extracts that have been recognised for centuries for their beautifying and health-restoring benefits. The minerals and trace elements in sea water are similar to those of blood plasma, and the body can absorb these minerals from water treatments via the skin, especially when water is heated to body temperature.

SEAWEED IS A VITAL INGREDIENT in thalassotherapy treatments. It is a rich source of iodine, a mineral that stimulates the thyroid gland to produce the hormone thyroxine, the primary regulator of the body's metabolism. Special thalassotherapy centres offer a variety of treatments, ranging from seaweed and sea water baths to sea mud body wraps. These treatments aim to boost circulation, eliminate toxins and alleviate fatigue.

WATER THERAPY, or hydrotherapy, is another treatment that involves the use of water, usually from a mineral spring. The treatments use varying water temperatures to treat the body; hot water is initially used to stimulate and has a secondary relaxing effect, while cold water invigorates and tones. Alternating hot and cold showers or baths peps up circulation, decongests the blood flow and revives body tissue. Jets of water help to pummel the body back into shape and boost circulation. Hydrotherapy is ideal for treating conditions ranging from sports injuries to skin disorders, as part of a detoxification programme or to reduce stress.

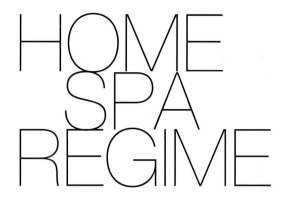

HOME SPA REGIME

Reap the benefits of a spa experience in the comfort of your own home. Allocate a day or weekend to pure indulgence and pamper yourself with treatments inspired by spa culture. Devise a schedule to suit you, take the phone off the hook and make your home a spa retreat.

FOOT TREAT

Treating your feet to a massage will benefit your whole body. Smooth oil or moisturiser onto the soles of your feet and knead them firmly with your thumbs, working from the outer edges to the centre of the soles in small, circular motions. Then massage the rest of your feet and ankles using your fingertips, working in sweeping, upward strokes.

RELAXATION

Take time out to relax completely – either have an afternoon nap, spend an hour reading or meditate. If you haven't meditated before, try this basic exercise: sit upright in a chair, place your hands on your lap, palms facing upwards, close your eyes and take deep breaths. Counting from 10 down, focus on relaxing each part of your body. Start with your head and work downward. By the time you reach one, your body should be completely relaxed and your mind free from any worries. Remain in this relaxed state for five minutes or longer.

HAIR PACK

Shampoo your hair and then treat it to a deep-conditioning hair pack. Alternatively, slather on your existing conditioner and wrap your hair in a hot towel for 10 minutes to step up the activity of the conditioner.

SALT GLOW

If you have bad circulation or need to deep-cleanse your body, a salt glow is the perfect treatment. Fill a cup with coarse sea salt and moisten it with water to form a sticky paste. Scoop a handful of the paste in each hand and massage it into your skin, starting at your feet and working up your body (avoiding the delicate bust and neck area). Use up-and-down or circular movements and try to create a good amount of friction. Rinse the salt off with warm water, vigorously towel-dry your skin and go to bed immediately. Don't be surprised if you sweat profusely, your body is shifting unwanted toxins. Avoid this treatment if you are diabetic and using insulin, or if you have cardiovascular problems or skin disorders.

HYDROTHERAPY BLITZ

Target problem zones on the hips and thighs with a high-powered shower jet. Work over your skin in circular motions with the shower nozzle to jump-start circulation and shift toxins. Alternate the water temperature from warm to cold for the maximum benefit.

EXERCISE

Incorporate an hour's out-door activity into your day. Go for a walk along the beach or in the park to boost your circulation and invigorate your body. Walk at a pace that leaves you feeling slightly breathless. For the maximum benefit, try pumping your arms backwards and forwards as you walk.

MUD MASK

They're messy to use, but mud masks are effective deep-cleansers, as they contain negatively charged ions that attract positively charged impurities. Sponge the mask onto damp skin, leave it on for the specified time and then rinse it off in the shower. While you're removing the mask, work over your body with a face-cloth to intensify the cleansing process.

SALTY SOLUTION

Consuming excess amounts of alcohol, caffeine and nicotine affects the body's metabolism, contributing to the formation of cellulite. Sea salts contain salt and seaweed extracts. They are a rich source of trace elements, including iodine, which is reputed to 'unblock' the metabolism. Soak in a warm bath with two cups of sea salt. To create the perfect ambience, listen to some soothing sounds and burn some aromatherapy oils or aromatic candles.

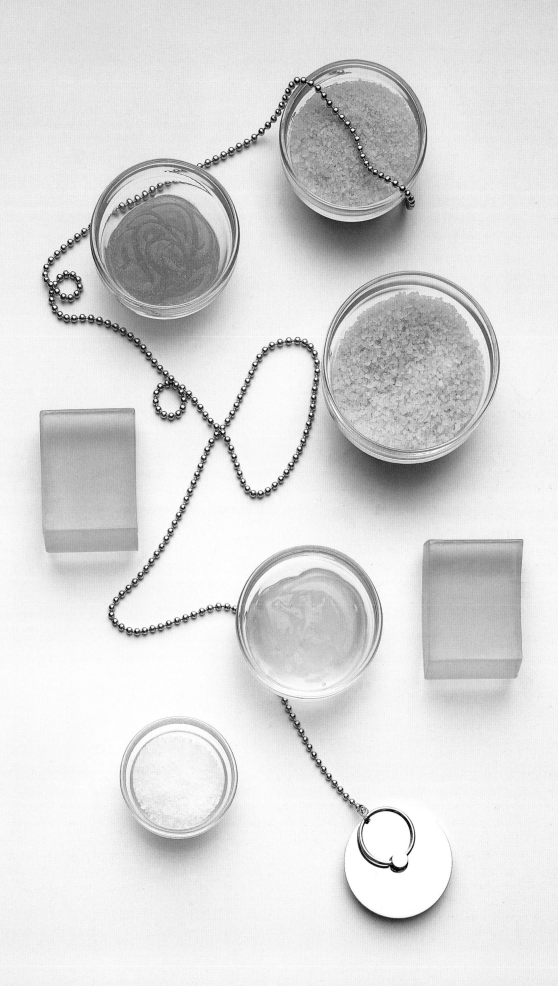

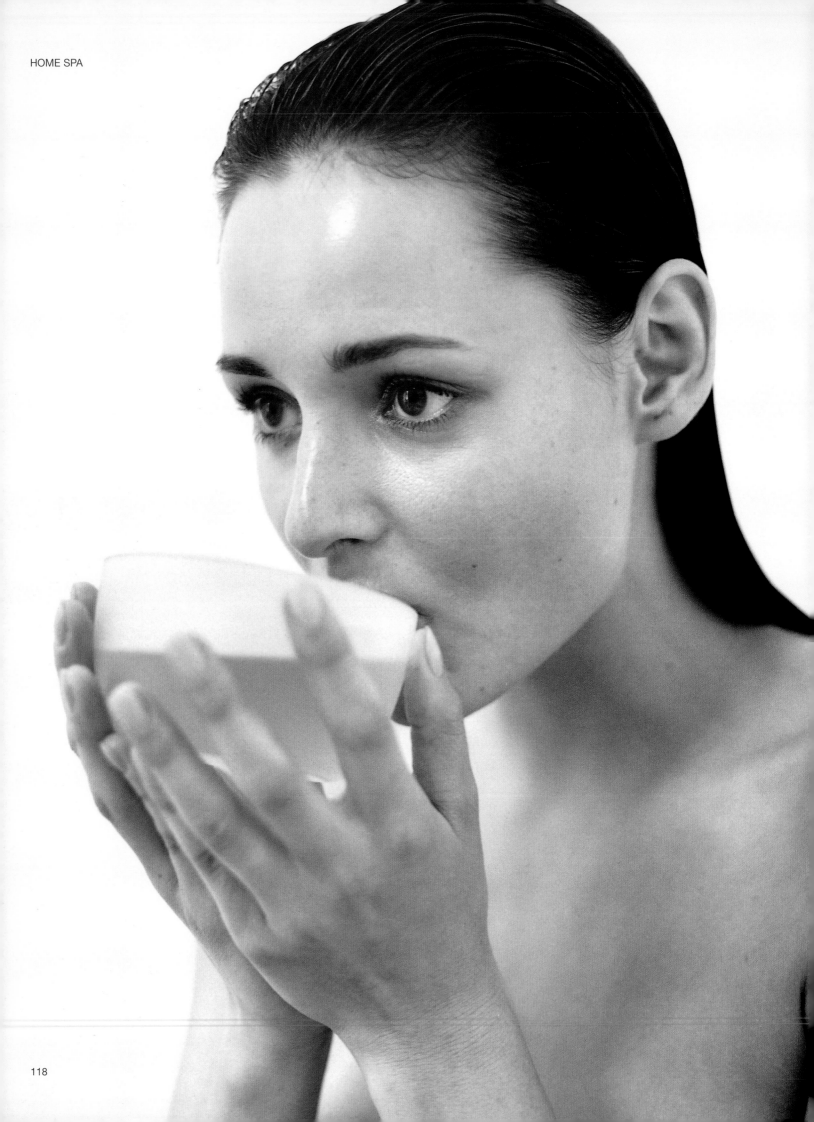

SPA CUISINE

Forget the idea that spa food has to be bland and insipid. To satisfy your palate, follow this eating plan and reap the benefits of nutritious low-fat, high-fibre meals.

BREAKFAST

Hotcakes with banana, berries and yoghurt

2 eggs
150g (5 oz) sugar
1½ cups (12 fl oz) skim milk
½ teaspoon vanilla essence
2½ cups self-raising flour, sieved
½ teaspoon bicarbonate of soda (baking soda)
2 tablespoons butter, melted
200g (7 oz) berries, such as raspberries and blueberries
2 teaspoons sugar
200g (7 oz) low-fat yoghurt
8–10 strawberries, crushed
1 banana, sliced
spray olive oil

To make the hotcake batter, whisk eggs, half the sugar, milk and vanilla essence together, then sprinkle in flour and bicarbonate of soda and mix. Melt the butter in a saucepan on low heat and whisk it into the flour mixture. Place the berries and the rest of the sugar in a saucepan over low heat, stirring occasionally. Heat a frypan or skillet and lightly spray it with olive oil. Add a spoonful of the batter mixture to the frypan or skillet and spread it into a 10cm (4 inch) circle. Cook the batter for two minutes, or until the surface of the hotcake begins to bubble. It is then ready to turn. Continue to cook for two minutes after turning, or until golden. To serve, place 2–3 hotcakes in the middle of a plate. Add banana slices on top, then a spoonful of the warm berry mixture (the juices will run over the sides of the cakes). Top with a spoonful of yoghurt mixed with the strawberries and serve immediately. Serves 2.

Couscous with poached fruit and cinnamon

½ cup (4 fl oz) water
¾ cup (6 fl oz) orange juice
2 tablespoons caster (superfine) sugar
1 teaspoon vanilla essence
1 cinnamon stick
4 apricots, dried
2 prunes, dried
2 dates, pitted
2 figs
2 handfuls sultanas
1 handful currants
¾ cup (6 fl oz) skim milk
½ cup (4 fl oz) couscous

Prepare the poached fruit the night before by mixing the water, orange juice, sugar, vanilla essence and cinnamon stick in a saucepan. Heat the mixture gently and bring to the boil. Add the fruit, then pour the mixture into a separate container, leave to cool and refrigerate overnight. To prepare the couscous, pour skim milk into a saucepan and bring to the boil. Add couscous and stir gently. Place the lid on the saucepan and leave the couscous to steam for 2–5 minutes. Meanwhile, warm the fruit mixture in a saucepan. To serve, spoon warm couscous into a bowl and pour the fruit and juice on top. Serves 2.

Asian breakfast

1 cup (8 fl oz) jasmine rice
sesame oil
2 eggs
soy sauce
1 handful sesame seeds, toasted
Optional spicy dressing
2 red chillies, sliced
1 teaspoon sugar
½ cup (4 fl oz) rice vinegar

Cook the rice until tender. Grease the inside of two 2½cm (1 inch) ramekins (ovenproof dishes) with sesame oil and break an egg into each dish. Place dishes in the microwave for 30 seconds at 1000 watts, or 40 seconds at 750 watts. The eggs will be soft in the centre (they shouldn't explode). To serve, place the rice in two bowls and then spoon the egg on top. Drizzle with soy sauce and sprinkle with sesame seeds. Serve immediately. For a spicy alternative, fry chillies, add sugar and rice vinegar, and use as a dressing. Serves 2.

LUNCH

Miso soup with noodles

spray olive oil
1 small carrot, grated
1 x 2–3cm (5–8 inch) piece
  ginger, grated
1 clove garlic, crushed
1 small onion, diced
1 celery stick, diced
500ml (18 fl oz) vegetable
  stock
500ml (18 fl oz) water
250g (9 oz) pre-cooked
  soba or buckwheat
  noodles
3 tablespoons dark miso
  paste mixed with ¼ cup
  (2 fl oz) water
soy or fish sauce to taste

Spray a saucepan with olive oil and sauté the carrot, ginger, garlic, onion and celery. Add the stock and water and simmer for 10 minutes. Add the noodles to the stock and water and bring to the boil. Stir in the miso paste and water, and simmer, without boiling, for two minutes. Taste soup and season with soy or fish sauce, then serve. Serves 2.

Nori rolls with red cabbage and sesame slaw

2 cups organic brown rice
½ cup (4 fl oz) rice vinegar
½ cup (4 fl oz) white sugar
¼ teaspoon salt
1 packet nori paper
  (Japanese seaweed,
  available from
  supermarkets or
  health food stores)
wasabi
1 small Lebanese
  cucumber, sliced
½ avocado, sliced
¼ red cabbage, sliced
  finely
2 shallots, peeled and
  diced
1 carrot, grated
1 cup bean shoots
2 tablespoons sesame
  seeds, toasted
½ cup (4 fl oz) low-fat
  yoghurt
30g (1 oz) pickled ginger
30ml (1 fl oz) sesame oil

Cook the rice until tender using the absorption method. Heat the rice vinegar, sugar and salt in a saucepan, stirring continuously until the sugar dissolves. Pour rice into a dish and add just enough of the heated liquid to coat the rice lightly. Cover the dish with a tea-towel and leave to cool. Place nori paper flat in front of you. (Have a small bowl of water within reach.) Wet your hands and shake off the excess water. Flatten handfuls of rice in a thin layer over the paper, leaving a 1cm (½ inch) strip clear at the top. Spread a small amount of wasabi over the rice a quarter of the way up the paper, then place the cucumber and avocado on the wasabi in thin strips. Roll the nori paper up, wetting the end of the paper to seal. You can also add tuna, salmon, bean shoots, carrot, marinated vegetables, or fried tofu. To make the sesame slaw, mix the red cabbage, bean shoots, shallots, carrot, sesame seeds, yoghurt, pickled ginger and sesame oil. To serve, slice the nori rolls with a wet knife and serve with the slaw. Serves 4.

Bruschetta with baba ghannouj, roast tomatoes, and marinated cucumbers

4 medium tomatoes
salt and cracked pepper
  to taste
1 teaspoon parsley,
  chopped
1 large eggplant
  (aubergine)
juice of half a lemon
1 clove garlic, crushed
2 teaspoons tahini
1 small Lebanese
  cucumber
½ teaspoon sugar
½ cup (4 fl oz) rice vinegar
4 x 2cm (1 inch) thick
  slices of Italian bread
spray olive oil
1 bunch rocket (arugula)
cracked pepper

Place the tomatoes on a non-stick baking tray, sprinkle with salt, pepper and half the parsley. Slow roast them at 100°C (210°F) for 60 minutes, or until tender. To make the baba ghannouj, pierce skin of the eggplant with a fork and place it under a hot grill until the skin blackens (this gives it a rich smoky flavour). Then bake it in the oven at 180°C (350°F) for 10–15 minutes. Remove it from the oven and leave to cool. When cool, peel off the black skin. Lightly blend eggplant, lemon juice and the rest of parsley, garlic, tahini, and salt and pepper. Season to taste. To prepare the cucumber, peel it using a peeler. Shave strips of cucumber with a peeler, place the strips in a bowl, sprinkle with sugar, and pour on the vinegar. Leave to stand for 15 minutes and drain just before serving. Lightly spray the bread with olive oil and place under a hot grill to toast. To serve, spread the baba ghannouj on the bread, then place the tomatoes, rocket leaves and cucumber on top. Sprinkle with cracked pepper and serve. Serves 2.

DINNER

Grilled fish with pumpkin and red capsicum salad

¼ pumpkin, skinned and diced into 2cm (1 inch) cubes
1 large capsicum, diced into 2cm (1 inch) cubes
spray olive oil
1 tablespoon wholegrain mustard
1 tablespoon lemon juice
2 tablespoons olive oil
salt and pepper to taste
2 pieces white fish, filleted
juice of 1 lemon (extra)
½ bunch rocket (arugula)
chives or shallots, chopped

Place the pumpkin and capsicum on a non-stick baking tray sprayed with olive oil and bake in the oven at 180°C (350°F) for 20 minutes, or until tender. To make the dressing, mix the mustard, lemon juice, olive oil, salt and pepper. Once capsicum and pumpkin are cooked, add the dressing. Cook the fish by splashing it with a little lemon juice, and placing it under a heated grill until the flesh flakes but is still moist. Serve by placing the rocket on top of the fish and sprinkle with chives or shallots to garnish. Serves 2.
Optional: this dish can also be served with steamed green vegetables.

Poached chicken with beetroot confit and green beans

spray olive oil
1 onion, diced
1 bunch fresh beetroot, grated
½ cup (4 fl oz) orange juice
¼ cup (2 fl oz) balsamic vinegar
¼ cup sugar
½ bunch of thyme, chopped
2 chicken breasts, skinned
1 clove garlic, crushed
salt and pepper to season
500ml (18 fl oz) chicken stock
200g (7 oz) whole green beans, washed and tailed

Spray a saucepan with olive oil and lightly sauté the onion until translucent. Add the beetroot and toss until warm. Add orange juice, vinegar, sugar and thyme. Stir well and simmer gently until beetroot is tender and liquid is absorbed. If the beetroot is not cooked sufficiently add a little more water. Rub the chicken with garlic, salt and pepper. Heat chicken stock in a saucepan and bring to the boil. Then reduce the heat and add the chicken. Gently poach the chicken on each side for five minutes or until it is cooked. Remove the chicken from the pan and cover with aluminium foil to keep warm. Steam the beans for five minutes. To serve, place two spoonfuls of beetroot on each plate and top with the whole beans. Slice the chicken breasts diagonally and place them on top of the beans. Dress with a little chicken stock, or sprinkle with balsamic vinegar. Serves 2.

Braised chinese vegetables and brown rice

1 cup brown rice
spray olive oil
1 bunch baby bok choy, quartered and washed
1 onion, sliced
1 x 4cm (2 inch) piece of ginger, grated
3 cloves garlic, crushed
150ml (5 fl oz) sweet soy
2 tablespoons soy sauce
juice of 1 lemon
2 tablespoons sesame oil
500ml (18 fl oz) chicken stock
100g (4 oz) oyster mushrooms
100g (4 oz) bean sprouts
100g (4 oz) fresh bamboo shoots
shallots or coriander, chopped, to garnish

Cook the rice until tender. Spray a large wok with olive oil, heat, and lightly sauté bok choy, onion, ginger and garlic until soft. Add the sweet soy, soy sauce, lemon juice, sesame oil and chicken stock. Bring to the boil. Then add oyster mushrooms, bean sprouts and bamboo shoots and heat through. To serve, place vegetables on a bed of rice and garnish with chopped shallots or coriander. Serves 2.

SPA LIVING

FOLLOW THESE STEPS TO ACHIEVE A HEALTHIER LIFESTYLE

LOOSE LEAVES

When you drink herbal teas, brew loose tea leaves (they have higher medicinal properties than the finely ground extracts used in tea bags). They may cost more but they can be used for three infusions – just top up your tea pot with hot water.

MAKING SENSE

Use essential oils as room fresheners. Sprinkle a few drops on the carpet, or on a light bulb or oil burner. Light an unscented candle and leave it to burn until a pool of melted wax forms. Then add two drops of your favourite essential oil.

EARLY FRUITS

Eating fresh fruit or raw vegetable juices until midday benefits the liver's elimination process, which is at its most active between midnight and midday. Consuming other foods during this period can interfere with this cleansing activity.

BEAUTY RITUAL

Japanese tradition involves cleansing with oil and water. Massage camelia oil into your face to dissolve make-up and dirt. Remove it with cotton wool, then use a wash-off cleanser. Rinse with warm water, then splash cold water over your face.

CUT OUT CAFFEINE

Like any stimulant, the effects of caffeine are short-lived and can cause exhaustion, nervousness, irritability, and headaches. Wean yourself off coffee (it takes at least four days to break the habit). Try drinking herbal teas or coffee substitutes.

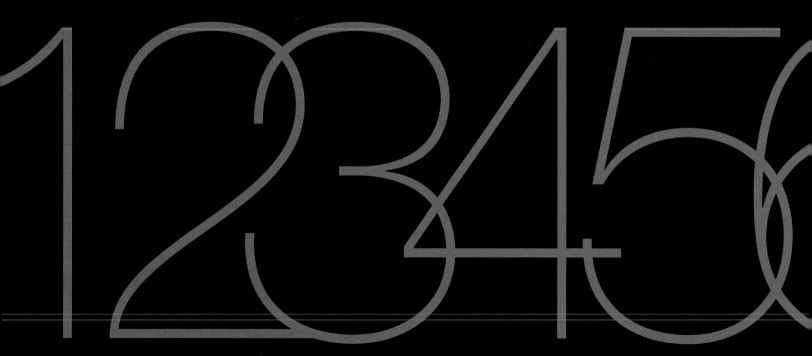

NATURAL BOOST

Aloe vera is known for its beautifying and cleansing properties. Aloe vera gel soothes sunburn and helps skin heal without scarring, while the juice (which is available from health food stores), is a potent natural cleanser and aids digestion.

COLD RELIEF

To relieve flu-like symptoms, add one drop each of lavender and tea-tree oil to 600ml warm water and breathe in the vapours. At night, put one drop each of lavender and eucalyptus oil on your pillowcase as a relaxant and decongestant.

LIVE CULTURE

Eating live natural yoghurt made with acidophilus helps to replace valuable bacteria in the gut, lost by ill-health and from antibiotics. It destroys harmful bacteria that can lead to bowel infections and can also be used to treat thrush.

CYSTITIS CURE

If you detect the onset of cystitis, treatment within the first three hours will prevent symptoms from setting in. Try taking powdered vitamin C diluted with water (available from health food stores) or drinking cranberry juice to neutralise urine.

HEALTHY SNACK

Eating strawberries is the perfect way to curb hunger pangs without piling on the pounds. Strawberries are a rich source of vitamin C, which enhances the body's ability to absorb iron from other foods and generally helps to cleanse the system.

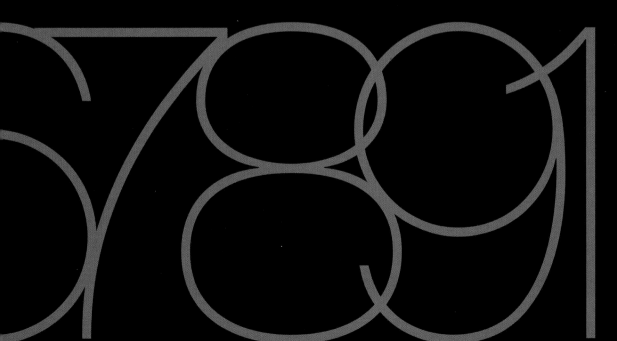
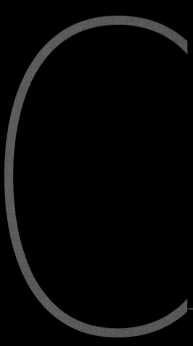

PROBLEM

Should you apply cold water to your body?

If you have a cold shower as a pick-me-up in the morning, warm your muscles first by having a warm shower or by exercising. Cold water on a cold body is too much of a shock to the system.

Can your body's water levels affect your energy reserves?

Your muscles contain a high concentration of water and some fatigue can be caused by dehydration, so make sure you always drink plenty of water.

How can you cope with anxiety?

When you're feeling anxious, munch on raw vegetables – the crunching motion releases tension.

Which aromatherapy oils should you burn to relax yourself?

Essential oils of jasmine, camomile, rose, lavender and marjoram all have calming properties.

Is there a quick fix to soothe aching muscles?

As a post–work-out treat, relax in a warm bath laced with a handful of Epsom salts. These draw out the lactic acid that builds up in muscles during exercise and can help prevent stiffness.

Is it worth drinking a fresh juice every day?

Incorporating a fresh fruit or vegetable juice into your daily diet, even if you're not undergoing a detox, will benefit your general health.

Can creams really shift stubborn patches of cellulite?

Cream won't remove cellulite – expensive preparations are a waste of time and money.

What's the best way to shave your legs?

Allow your hair to absorb water for at least three minutes while in the shower or bath. This causes the hair to swell, which makes it easier to remove.

Can the weather affect how you feel?

Research confirms that your white blood cell count varies with the seasons. During humid weather more people suffer from migraines and fluctuating temperatures affect blood pressure.

How can you ensure a peaceful night's sleep?

Steer clear of alcohol, caffeine and nicotine for at least four hours before retiring to bed.

SOLUTION

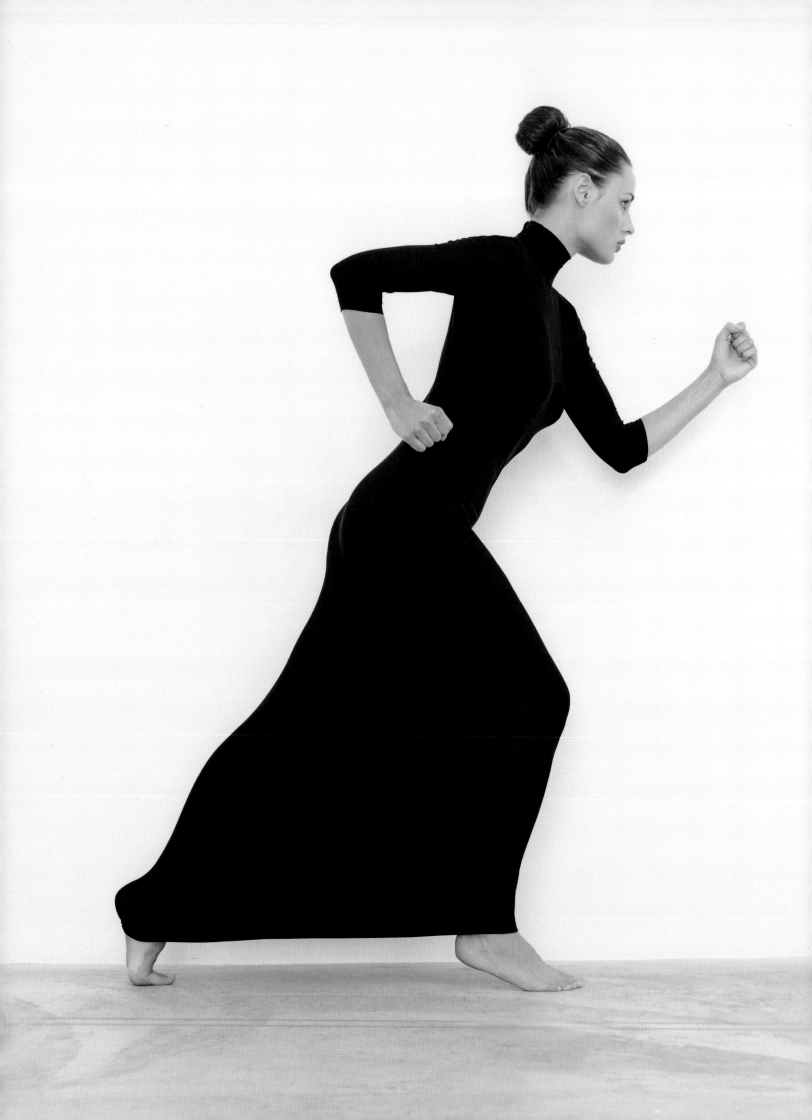

EXERCISE

Exercise regularly to improve your physique and to sustain your general health. Incorporate physical activity into your lifestyle so that you can enjoy its many benefits.

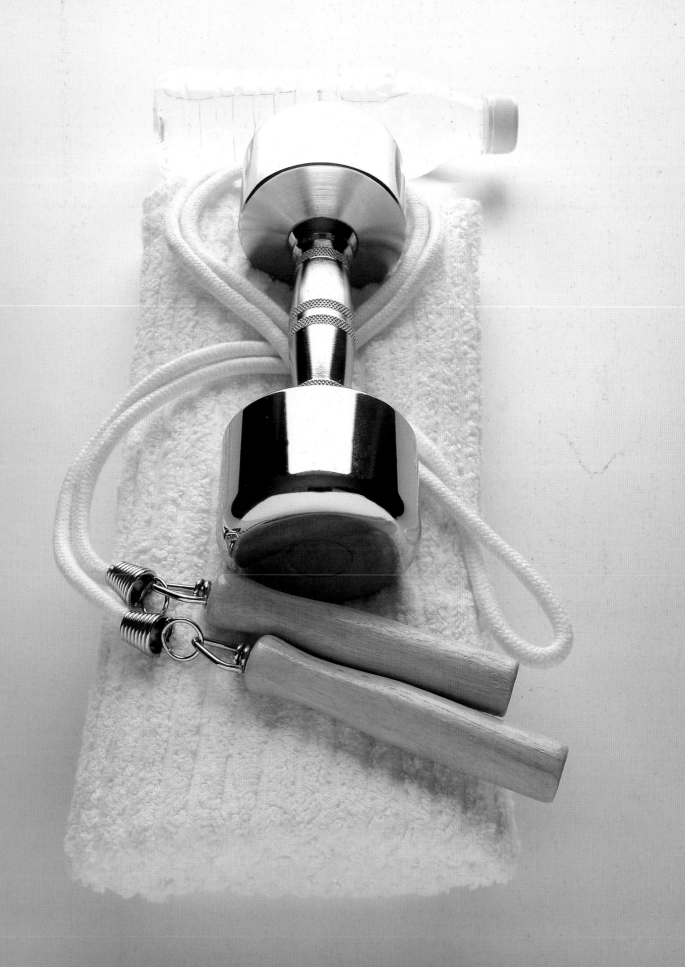

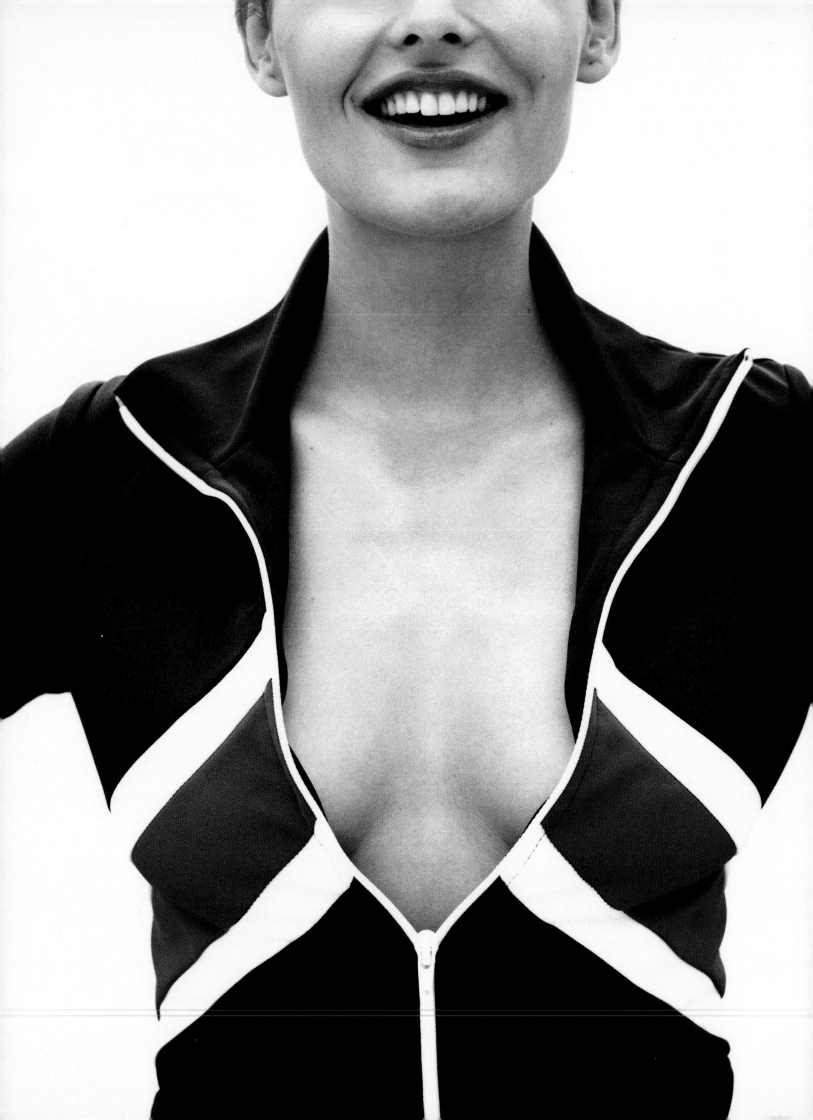

FITNESS HIGH

Apart from keeping you flexible, strong and lean, regular exercise provides a long-lasting feel-good factor. Exercise stimulates the body's pituitary gland to release natural opiates known as endorphins. This is why you experience a 'natural high' when you work out.

BECOMING FIT USED TO MEAN gruelling workouts and endless weights sessions. The accepted wisdom today is that fitness can be achieved by taking part in enjoyable recreational sports.

THE SECRET TO SUCCESSFUL BODY SHAPING lies in combining different types of exercise. Aerobic exercise, which increases the body's intake of oxygen, increases stamina and maintains a healthy cardiovascular and respiratory system. Aerobic activities, such as brisk walking, dancing, cycling and jogging, also stimulate the metabolism, creating energy from the body's fats and carbohydrates. Fats can only be converted into energy in the presence of oxygen, which is why aerobic activity is ideal for maintaining body weight. Muscle-toning activities such as yoga or stretching complement aerobic exercise, as they improve flexibility and overall strength.

BODY WORK

Devise an exercise program that is specifically suited to your body shape and follow these guidelines to accentuate your best traits and balance your overall shape:

ECTOMORPHS are typically tall with slender, long limbs, usually with a lean torso and small breasts. Concentrate on building overall muscle tone and opt for low-impact aerobics to improve cardiovascular fitness. Body sculpting classes will make your figure more curvaceous. Avoid going for the burn – you can't afford to lose calories. Skating, walking, rollerblading, swimming, Tai Chi and stretch classes will all be beneficial.

ENDOMORPHS are characterised by a small, round build that is usually pear-shaped. Working the lower body, concentrating on the buttocks and thighs, will benefit this body shape. Try to burn calories to minimise curves and avoid training with heavy weights – you don't need to increase muscle mass. Suitable sports include low-intensity aerobics, yoga, stretching, skipping, running, horse-riding and cycling.

MESOMORPHS are usually voluptuous with large bones and well-developed limbs and lower body. Concentrate on aerobic exercise to burn calories and balance your lower and upper body. Improve your overall flexibility and muscle tone without bulking up. For the best results, try yoga, rowing, skipping, jogging, Pilates (see page 101) and body sculpting classes.

EXPERT ADVICE

Thirty minutes of aerobic activity three times a week reduces body fat and relieves depression.

Muscle-toning and strength training twice a week will help to prevent the muscle and bone loss that occurs with age. This inevitable process starts during your 20s and 30s.

Stretching regularly prevents injury and eliminates lower back pain.

Warm up first, cool down before stopping and if you're new to exercise, see a doctor before starting a fitness regime.

Aim to exercise at least three times a week for half an hour.

Exercise within your ability. Consult a personal trainer to evaluate your target zone (the safe rate for your heart-beat while exercising). Exercising at a rate above your target zone is detrimental to your health. If you exercise below this rate, you won't reap the full benefits of any kind of aerobic activity.

SPORTING ACTIVITY

SWIMMING

Swimming is perfect for maintaining overall body tone. Backstroke tightens the abdominal muscles, tones the legs and upper arms and burns the most kilojoules (2100–3360 [500–800 calories] per hour); freestyle improves body alignment and is beneficial for the cardio-vascular system; breast stroke strengthens the upper arms and works the inner thighs (avoid this stroke if you are pregnant, it puts additional strain on the base of the spine). Aim to swim for 20 minutes three times a week and alternate strokes for the best results.

REBOUNDING

Bouncing on a special rebounder (mini trampoline) is a fun way to get into shape. Rebounding offers the same benefits as other aerobic sports but, in addition to the cardiovascular benefits, the continual gravity/non-gravity activity of bouncing up and down stimulates the skin's cellular activity and the transportation of waste materials via the lymphatic system to waste disposal sites around the body. Rebounding can be done while watching television or listening to music – it is an easy activity to incorporate into your life.

DANCING

Any form of dance will improve all-round fitness. Controlled dance forms such as ballet improve muscle tone, strength and posture while high-energy movement gets the blood flowing, the heart pumping and burns calories.

YOGA

In addition to its mind/spirit benefits, yoga improves your body's flexibility and suppleness. Various poses stretch and strengthen the muscles and ligaments, stimulate circulation and massage the internal organs. It's a great way to maintain general health, balance the body and improve your inner calm. Yoga is also an effective technique for stress management.

CYCLING

Cycling improves co-ordination and muscle strength and is a great way to tone the lower half of the body. Fifteen minutes of cycling at a medium pace has the potential to burn 440–945 kilojoules (105–225 calories). For the best results, avoid cycling in areas that are polluted, congested with traffic, or pedestrians, or around traffic signals that require you to stop (cycling continuously is far more beneficial than stopping and starting). Ensure the seat and handle bars are in the correct position to prevent back strain.

SKIPPING

Skipping is a great way to tone the thighs, calves and buttocks. It improves aerobic endurance and also strengthens the back and shoulder joints. Aim to skip for 5–10 minutes each day. Start slowly and gradually build up your pace.

TENNIS

Tennis strengthens your lower body and shoulders, and improves your cardio-vascular system. Fifteen minutes of tennis has the potential to burn 380–500 kilojoules (90–120 calories).

JOGGING

Jogging and running are great circulation boosters. They also help keep your legs and thighs in trim and maintain overall fitness. (Avoid this type of activity if you have weak knees or ankles.) To avoid additional pressure on your joints, try not to jog or run on concrete pavements or hard ground.

POWER WALKING

Walking briskly is one of the most beneficial forms of activity. Fifteen minutes of fast walking can burn up to 315 kilojoules (75 calories). For the maximum benefit, keep your back straight, hold your stomach in and keep your buttocks taut. While walking, swing your arms, sway your hips and breathe in through your nose and out through your mouth. Avoid walking in heavily polluted areas.

TAI CHI

This Chinese martial art is a gentle way to tone your body and fine-tune your mind–body connection. Based on a series of slow, rhythmic poses that energise you through balance, control and breathing, Tai Chi is beneficial for stress, high blood pressure and heart complaints, as well as mental and physical alertness.

AQUA AEROBICS

Your body weighs 90% less in water, yet water resistance training is 12 times more effective than air resistance training, so working out in the water improves muscle tone and strength much faster than out-of-pool activities. You can do aqua aerobics classes, or alter-natively, try these simple exercises in the sea or in a pool. Stand with your body immersed in water to the top of your shoulders and jog on the spot, pumping the arms backwards and forwards for five minutes. Stand up straight, kick one leg out in front of you and lower it 15 times. Do the same with the other leg. To work your arms, stand with your feet shoulder-width apart, extend your arms at shoulder height in front of you with palms facing downward. Slowly sweep your arms back-wards and forwards, vertically. Repeat 15 times.

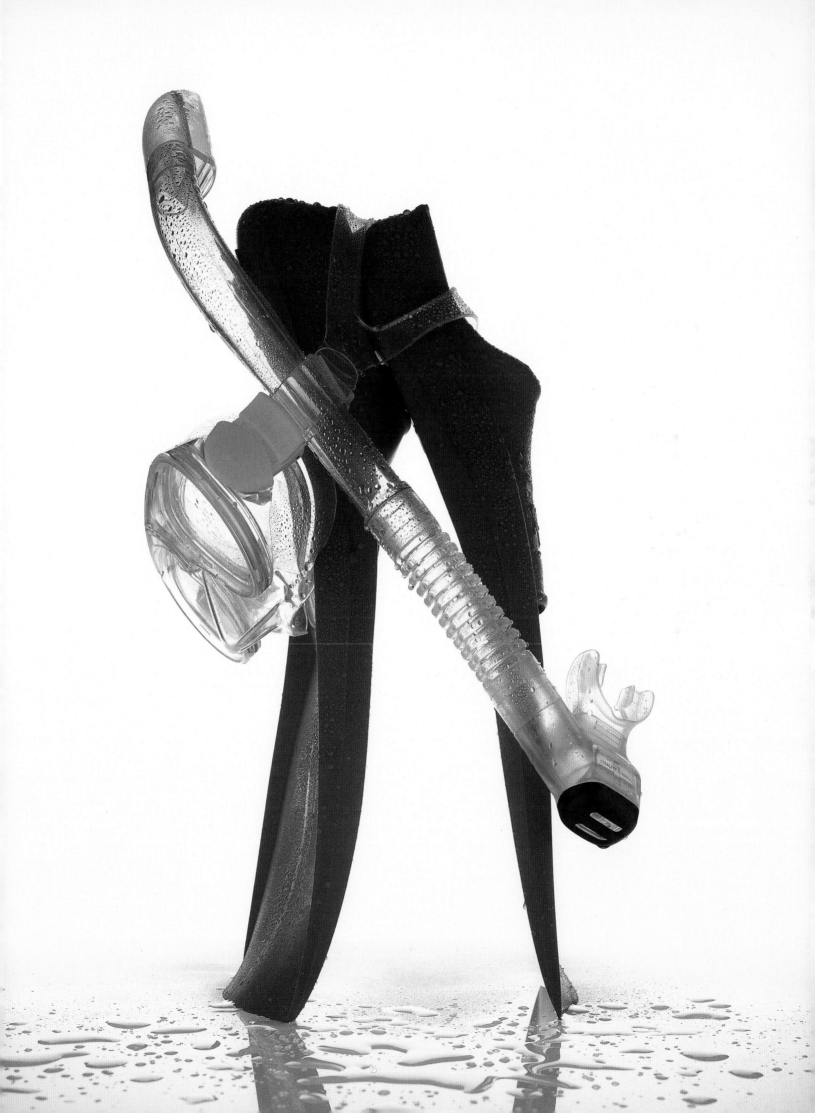

SPORTING SENSE

FOLLOW THESE STEPS TO ENHANCE YOUR WORK-OUT

CHANGE SPORTS

Boredom is a common reason for people to abandon an exercise regime and become unfit. Vary the type of activity you do to keep interested. Try one of the many recreational sports or exercise with a friend to maintain your motivation.

CALORIE BURNERS

If you don't have time to exercise, think about the calories you burn doing chores that you probably hate. Half an hour of household cleaning, 16 minutes of scrubbing floors and 38 minutes of vacuuming each have the potential to burn 420 kilojoules (100 calories).

SALTY ANSWER

If you sweat a lot during exercise, there's no need to increase your salt intake: your diet will supply enough salt and your body will readjust to compensate for the loss – it conserves salt levels by reducing the concentration of salt in sweat and urine.

ENERGY ESSENCE

A pre-sport spritz of a cooling essence can improve your athletic performance. Menthol and eucalyptus have an energising effect: inhaling them stimulates the trigeminal nerve in the nose and palate, which in turn boosts your energy levels.

ENHANCE ABILITY

Before playing sports that require concentration, such as tennis or golf, inhale rosemary, basil, peppermint, ginger or juniper oil. These aromas send you into an 'alpha-wave' state (the deep concentration essential for optimum performance).

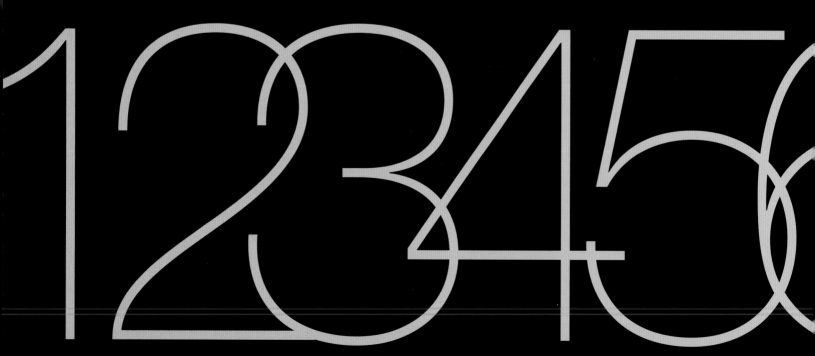

STRETCH WORK

Stretch for five minutes before and after exercise. Pre–work-out stretching warms the muscles. Post–work-out stretching prevents aching. Hold each stretch for 10–30 seconds. Never force a stretch and if it hurts, stop immediately.

FOOD THOUGHT

Don't overlook your diet: well-fuelled muscles work much more efficiently. Aim to eat nutritious, balanced meals that contain 60% carbohydrates, 20% protein and 20% fat. Increase your intake of raw vegetables and fresh fruits.

RUB DOWN

After a work-out, treat overworked muscles to an aromatic rub down. Blend two drops each of eucalyptus, peppermint and ginger oil with 15ml almond oil. Massage the blend into your body, working over aching muscles with kneading movements.

INJURY RELIEF

If you suffer from a sports injury, apply ice to the area for 20 minutes. Crush some ice and put it in a plastic bag, wrap two towels around it and place over the injury. Rest for 20 minutes and add ice again. Repeat this for three to four hours.

SHOCK ABSORB

When you work out, it is vital you wear the right sports shoes. For running, buy trainers with a high-density sole to absorb the powerful impact of your feet hitting the ground. Otherwise, you could damage your knees or Achilles tendons.

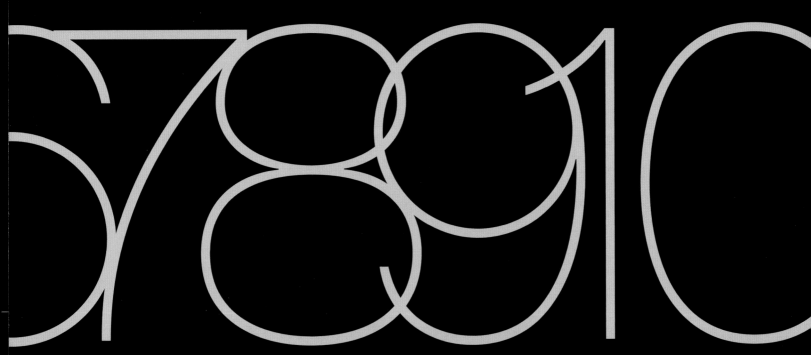

PROBLEM

Will wearing sunscreen while exercising block your pores?
Wearing sunscreen while you work out won't clog your pores or hinder sweating, it will actually have a cooling effect on your body.

Do you take iron tablets to counteract fatigue but still feel tired?
Try taking iron tablets every second day – sometimes the body blocks the absorption of iron if it is taken too frequently.

What's the best way to avoid dehydrating while exercising?
Fitness experts recommend that you should drink two glasses of fluid two hours before exercise, and sip water every 15–20 minutes during exercise.

If you suffer from hunger pangs before a work-out, what can you eat?
Snack on a banana at least 30 minutes before you exercise.

Is there a way to fake a great beach body?
Steer clear of carbohydrates before heading to the beach, they can bloat your stomach.

Are there foods your body needs if you exercise regularly?
Exercise increases your body's need for protein. Step up your intake of cereals, cheddar cheese, fish, fruit and vegetables, milk and soy products and nuts.

What are the best sporting activities to tone a sagging butt?
In-line skating, mountain biking and step aerobics will help keep your buttocks in shape.

What can you do if you have a serious aversion to exercise?
Set yourself realistic goals. Start off by making minor changes to your lifestyle, for example, walk up stairs instead of using lifts and stop using your car and walk.

What's an effective way to keep muscles toned?
Always work opposing muscle groups. If you work your triceps, work your biceps as well.

What is the best time of day to work out if you want to lose weight?
Some experts believe that exercising first thing in the morning is best if you want to shed a few pounds, because you burn fat stores faster on an empty stomach.

SOLUTION

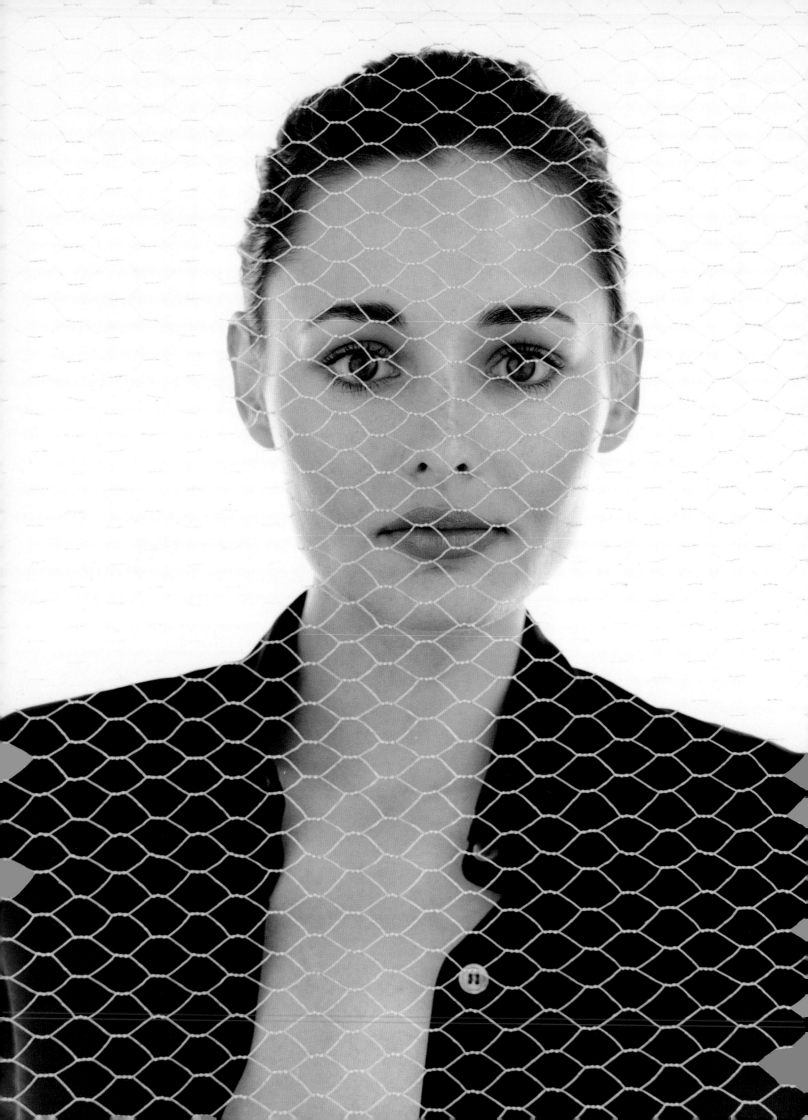

SURVIVAL

SURVIVING THE HARMFUL EFFECTS OF POLLUTION AND ULTRAVIOLET RADIATION IS THE REALITY OF MODERN LIVING. TAKE STEPS TO PROTECT YOURSELF AND ENJOY A HEALTHIER EXISTENCE.

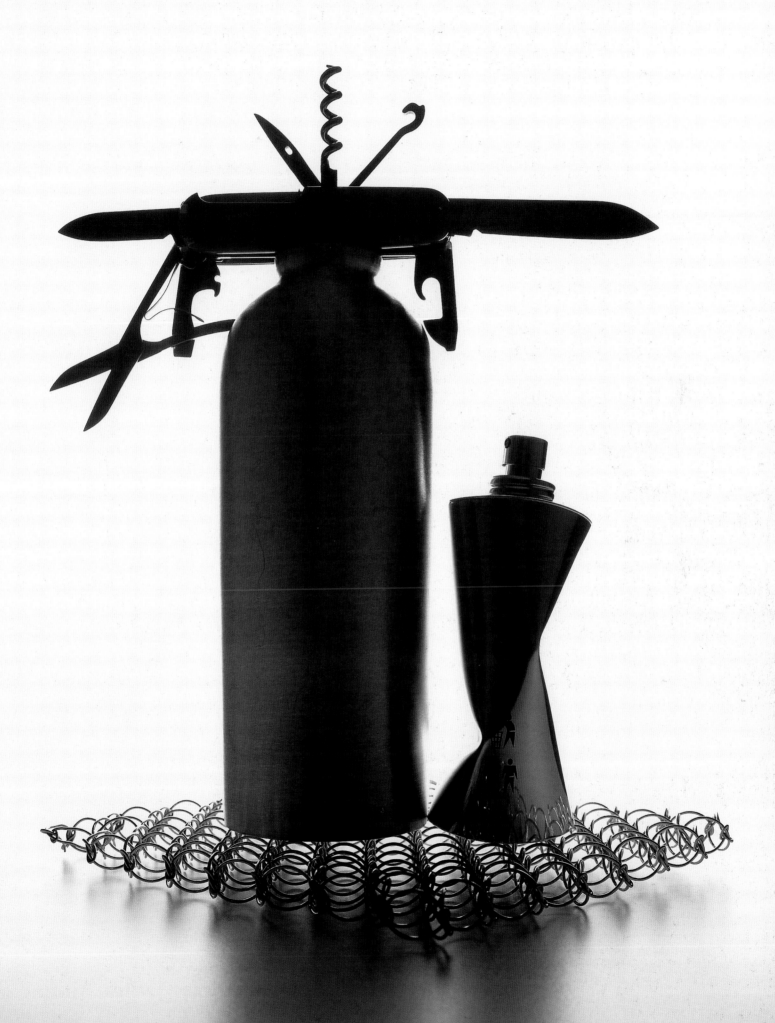

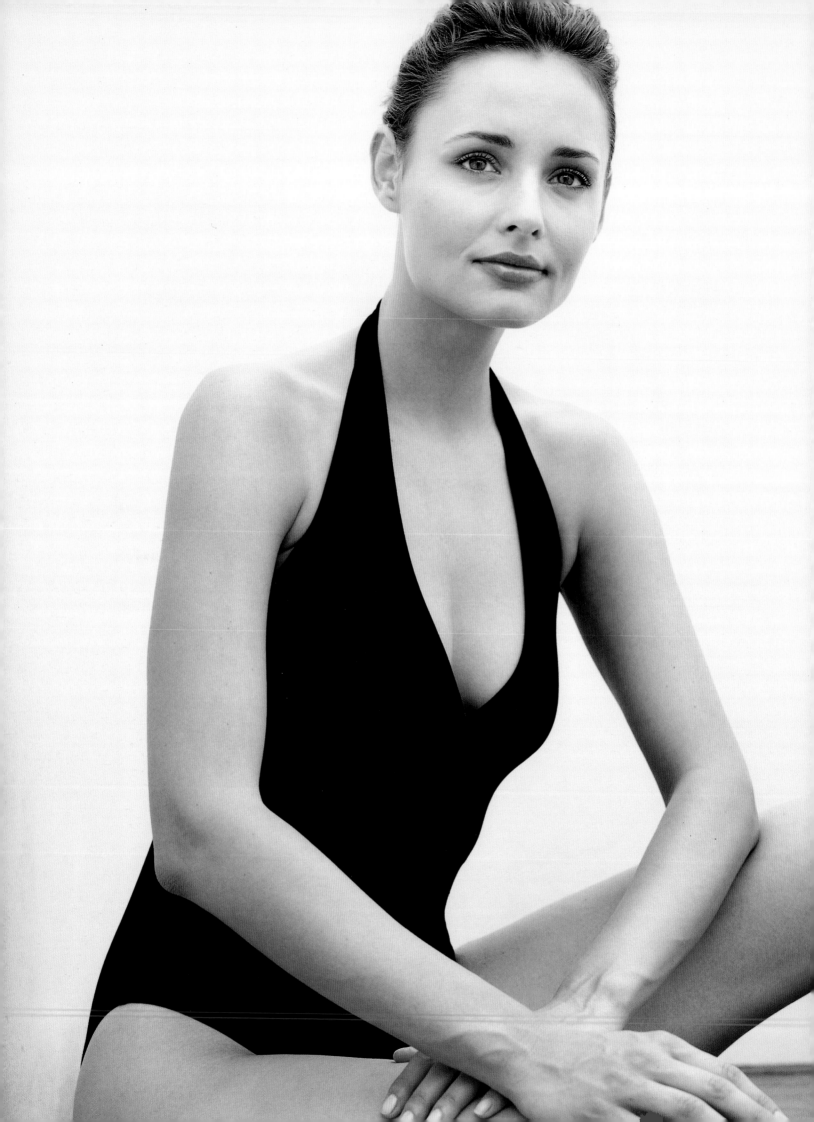

TOXIC LIVING

An increase in negative external factors, accelerated by the deterioration of the environment and modern lifestyles (stress, poor diet and lack of sleep), have made you a prime target for toxin assault. Invisible aggressors invade daily life: apples could be coated with pesticides, the paint on your walls could be poisoning you, and ingredients in cosmetics could be doing you more harm than good.

IF YOU HAVE A HEALTHY IMMUNE SYSTEM, efficient organs of elimination, and effective circulation and nervous systems, you may actually be able to cope with a large amount of toxicity. However, exposure to excessive amounts of toxins can lead to bioaccumulation (a build-up of foreign substances in the body), and disrupt the functioning of your organs.

UNDER ATTACK

When the body encounters toxins, whether from foods or pollution, it increases free radical activity. Each healthy cell receives at least 10 000 damaging 'hits' from these molecules every day. A certain amount of free radical activity is needed to kill bacteria and germs, but problems arise when the body produces too many and the process gets out of control.

FREE RADICALS ARE LARGELY the by-product of oxidation (the same process that causes cars to rust). They are also created by a number of external agents, including pollution, pesticides, tobacco, smoke, car fumes and ultraviolet light. Research suggests that free radicals can accelerate premature ageing and are also a major contributory factor in at least 50 of our most prevalent diseases, including coronary heart disease and can-

FIGHTING BACK

Antioxidants function as the body's main chemical defence against free radicals. Some antioxidants, such as oestrogen, the main female hormone, are made by the body, while others, such as vitamins E and C and beta-carotene (the precursor of vitamin A) are found in foods and cosmetic preparations. All antioxidants work in slightly different ways, but the overall effect is to mop up free radicals as they form and prevent them from doing serious damage within the body.

THERE IS STILL GREAT DEBATE over which is more effective, taking antioxidants orally or applying them topically. Both have their place. Antioxidants in beauty creams protect the skin from environmental factors, while antioxidants in tablets or foods help to neutralise the by-products of oxidation in the body.

SURVIVAL TACTICS

Start drinking green tea.
It's a natural source of antioxidants, which reputedly boost the immune system and strengthen the skin's defence mechanism, as well helping to prevent tooth decay and cancer. Research has shown that green tea has stronger effects on free radicals than vitamins C or E.

Drinking red wine in moderation
can actually benefit your health. The grapes used in red wine contain powerful anti-oxidants, known as procyanadins, which protect the body internally.

Take echinacea, a native
American herb best known for warding off colds and flu. It is also gaining favour as an anti-ageing remedy due to its antibiotic and immune-enhancing properties.

Half of the foods you eat should
be fresh fruits and raw vegetables. When consumed in their natural state, they are rich in antioxidants.

SURVIVAL TACTICS

If you have sensitive, allergy-prone skin, use sunscreens with physical filters. They will cause minimal irritation.

Smooth on a sunscreen before heading to the beach. Otherwise, the sun's rays will damage unprotected skin en route.

Protect your hair during sun exposure, as ultraviolet light has a drying effect and can cause colour to fade.

Always wear sunglasses which comply with the standard Eye Protection Factor, as eyes are prone to melanomas and cataracts.

During sporting activity, use a water-resistant or waterproof sunscreen. It will remain effective if you sweat or if you are exercising in water.

SUN EXPOSURE

The sun is one of our most deadly enemies. Any exposure to ultraviolet light, whether it causes a tan, sunburn or no visible reaction at all, prompts cellular damage that leads to, at the very least, signs of ageing, and at worst, skin cancer. The sun's light waves are categorised by their intensity:

ULTRAVIOLET A (UVA) have the longest wavelength and they penetrate into the skin's deepest layer, the dermis. Here they disturb the production of collagen and elastin, activate damaging free radicals and accelerate skin ageing.

ULTRAVIOLET B (UVB) rays only penetrate the skin's upper layer, the epidermis and they are responsible for skin cancers, allergies and sunburn. When skin is sunburnt, fluid leaks between the cells, causing swelling. The skin reddens as the blood capillaries dilate in an attempt to rid the skin of excess heat. Skin that has been burnt six times faces double the risk of developing fatal melanoma.

ULTRAVIOLET C (UVC) rays are the most damaging, but do not reach us because they are filtered by the ozone layer. However, there is growing concern about exposure to these rays with the thinning of the ozone layer.

INFRA-RED (IR) light is felt as heat and inflames cells, disrupts the skin's support network of collagen and elastin and damages the body's immune system.

THERE ARE TWO TYPES OF SUN-PROTECTION FILTERS in sunscreen products that screen out the sun's damaging wave-lengths. Products contain either physical or chemical filters, or a combination of both.

PHYSICAL FILTERS SIT ON THE SKIN'S SURFACE and reflect, rather than absorb, ultraviolet rays. Titanium dioxide and zinc oxide are the physical filters used in most sunscreens. They repel radiation at all wavelengths (including infra-red waves), which is essential as cancer and ageing involve the interaction of all wavelengths at varying degrees.

CHEMICAL FILTERS ABSORB ULTRAVIOLET LIGHT like a sponge and prevent the sun's rays from penetrating and attacking the skin. The fact that they can be mixed into any base, dissolved in gels, lotions, moisturising cream bases and waterproof formulations make them cosmetically acceptable.

THE SUN-PROTECTION FACTOR (SPF) of a product refers to the length of time you can remain in the sun safely. To calculate this protection time, multiply the SPF by the number of minutes you can stay in the sun unprotected without burning. For example, if your skin normally takes 10 minutes of sun exposure before starting to go red, using a sunscreen with SPF 15 will theoretically extend this to 150 minutes.

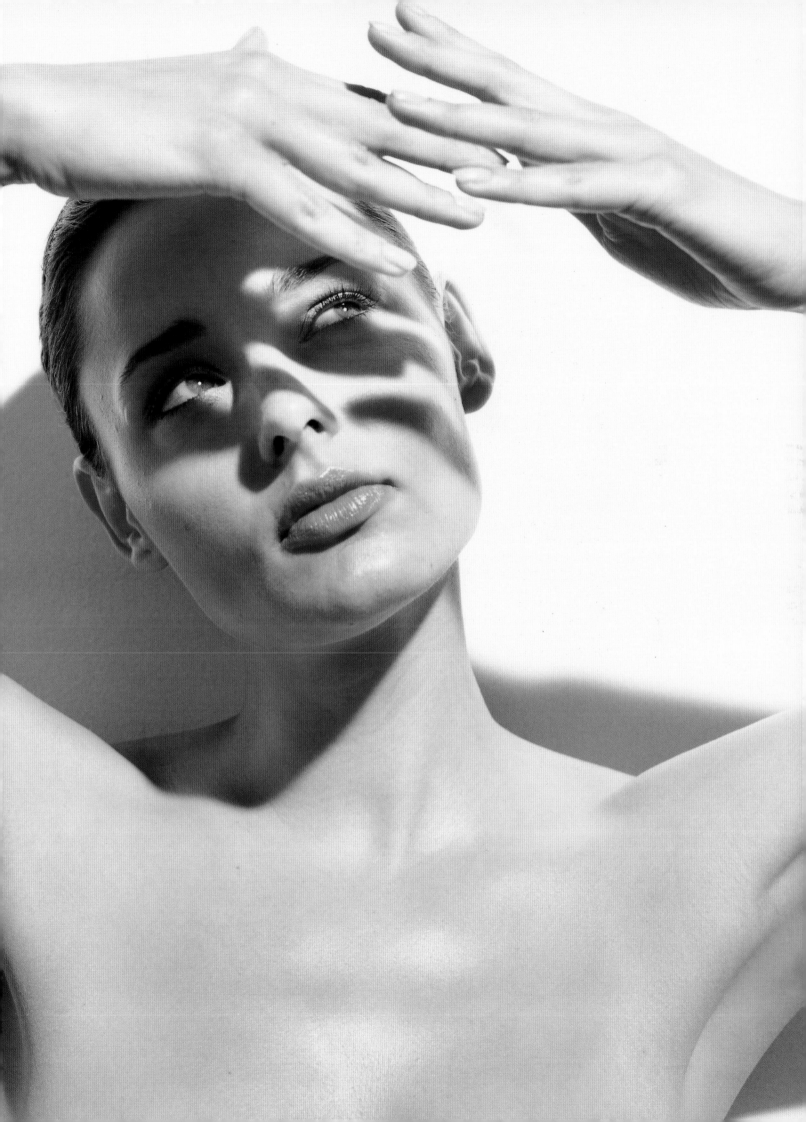

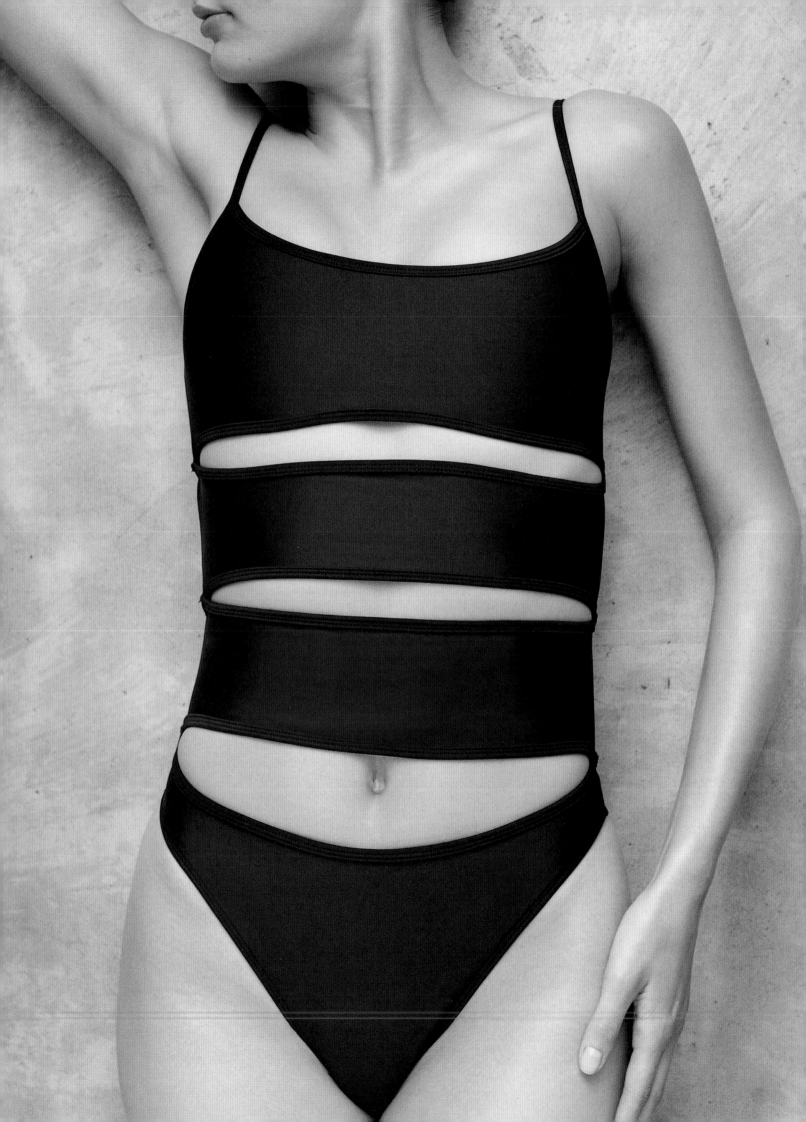

SUN SAFETY

PROTECTIVE CLOTHING

In the past, the only kinds of clothing that offered protection from ultraviolet rays were heavy, dark-coloured garments. Now a colourless dye with UV-absorbing properties is being used to sun-proof fabrics, giving them an SPF-equivalent of up to 50. Always wear a hat while in the sun and cover up at the beach to prevent sunburn.

FINDING THE FORMULA

Sun-protection products come in different formulations ranging from gels to creams, lotions and alcohol-based preparations. Look for a product most suited to your skin type. If you have an oily, problem complexion, use a gel formulation with physical filters. If you have dry skin, steer clear of alcohol- or gel-based sunscreens, which can aggravate dryness. A cream or lotion will be beneficial for its moisturising properties.

TAKE COVER

Stay out of the sun between 11am and 3pm when the sun is at its strongest and deadliest. Protect your skin even when it's overcast, as damaging ultraviolet rays penetrate clouds.
If small, white patches appear on your upper body after sun exposure, the cause could be a common yeast infection called pityriasis versicolor. The organism is present on everyone, but during sun exposure it may change and produce a chemical which disables the pigment-producing cells. To correct the problem, apply an anti-dandruff shampoo to the affected area while in the shower once a week for six weeks. Alternatively, the condition can be treated with a course of antibiotics. Seek advice from your doctor or dermatologist.

MOLE PATROL

Examine yourself regularly for any suspicious-looking freckles, moles or skin irregularities. Pay special attention to moles that have changed in shape or size, feel itchy, tender, painful, or are inflamed or bleeding. Always have any abnormalities checked out by the experts. If you detect cancerous moles in the early stages, they can be treated quickly and easily.

SELF-TANNING

One of the easiest ways to improve the appearance of your body is to give it an all-over radiant glow. Exposure to ultraviolet light is so damaging that the safest way to achieve colour is to fake it. Forget a session on the sunbed – artificial tanning beds are as lethal as the sun (they increase the risk of developing the deadliest form of skin cancer by seven times) – and opt for a self-tanning preparation.

FAKING A TAN HAS BECOME AN ART FORM. You can now determine the exact degree of colour you require, as the level of dihydroxyacetone, the active ingredient in the product which creates the colour, also dictates the depth of tone. Choose from light, medium and dark varieties. Products are easy to use and fast working. The results last for up to five days and you can prolong colour with regular top-up applications.

PRODUCT SELECTION

When choosing a self-tanning product, take your skin type into account. Moisture-rich cream formulas are best for dry skins; lotions suit normal and combination skins, as they are light and offer hydration without overloading the skin; and gels are ideal for oily skins, as they don't clog the pores. Look for a self-tanning preparation enriched with an alpha hydroxy acid complex, which improves the activity of the tanning ingredients.

APPLICATION

To apply a self-tanning preparation, first exfoliate your skin using a gentle, non-abrasive scrub to avoid irritation. Then massage the tanning product into the skin, blending thoroughly. During application, pay particular attention to dry areas such as the elbows, knees and ankles. After smoothing the preparation on, blot these areas with a tissue to remove any excess product that might create uneven colour.

IF YOU USE FAKE TAN ON YOUR FACE, pay close attention to the areas around your eyebrows and hairline because the active ingredient in the tanning product can discolour your hair. One way to avoid this is to slick Vaseline through your brows before the bronzing process.

ALWAYS WASH YOUR HANDS immediately after applying fake tan and if your palms are discoloured, soak them in lemon juice and then give them a gentle scrub with a nail brush.

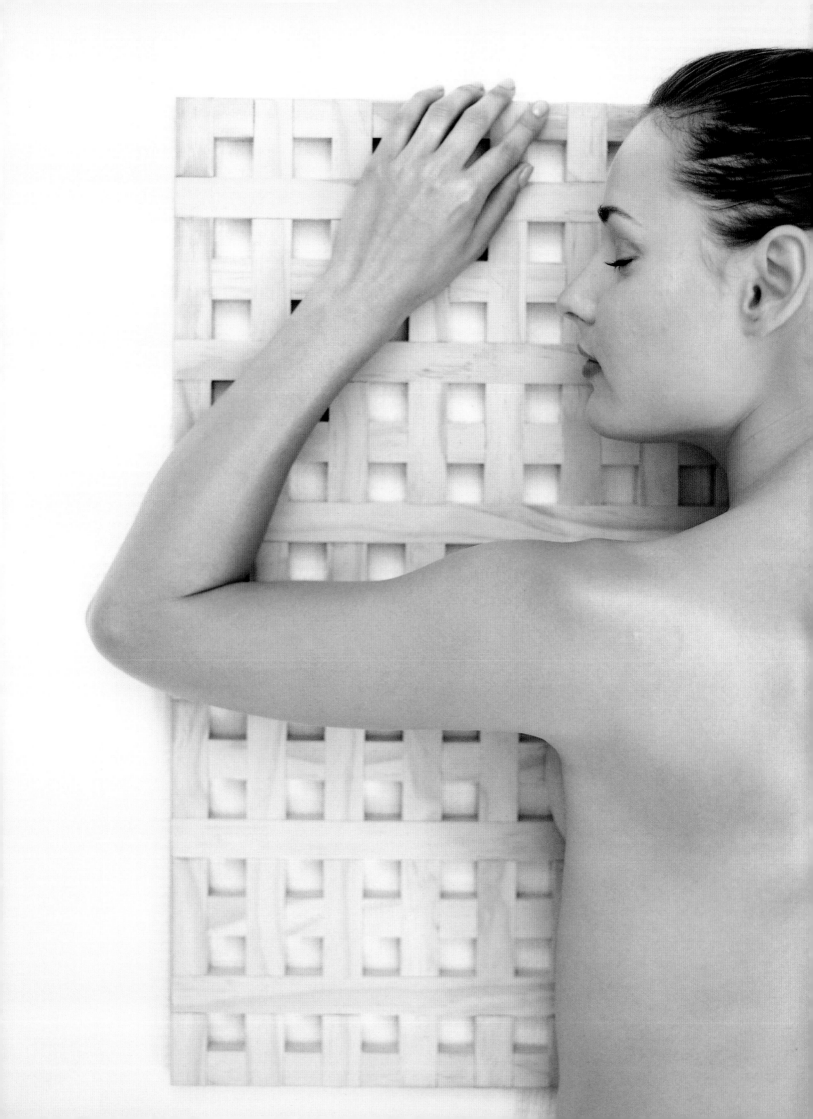

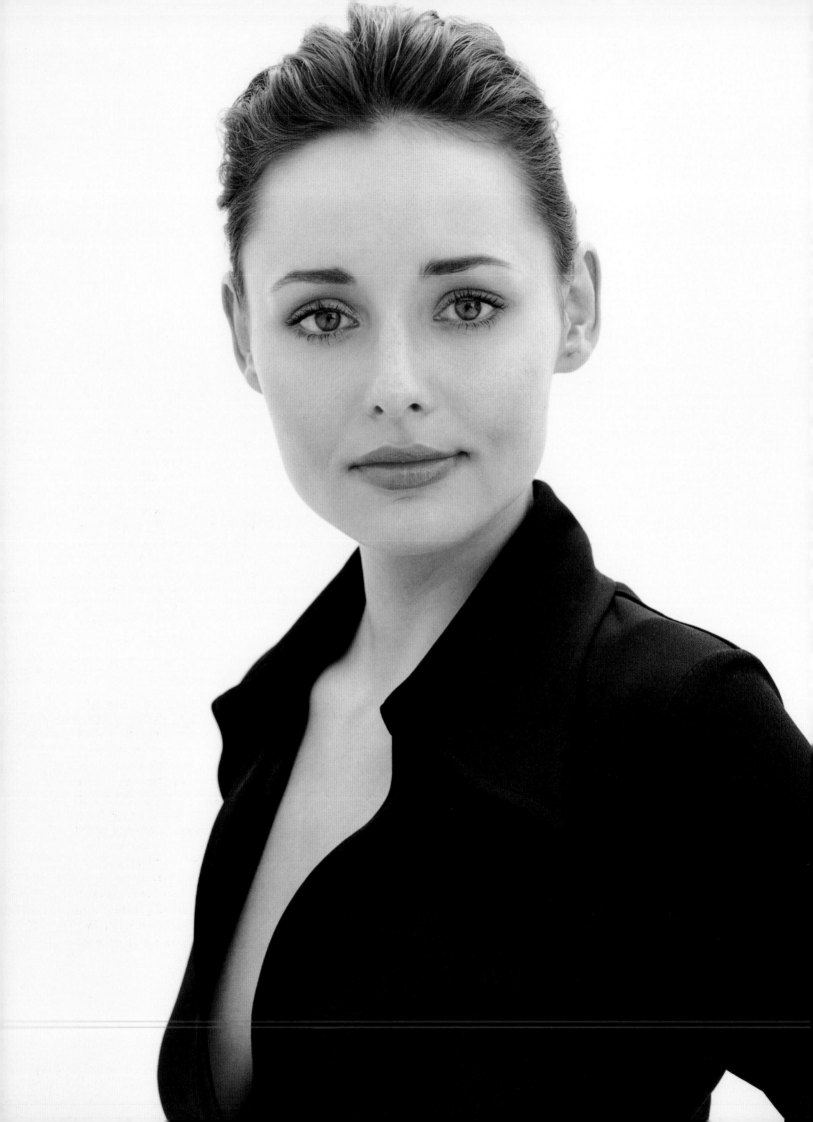

TOXIC OFFENDERS

Address the factors that assault you on a daily basis. Everything from cigarette smoke to the waves generated from computers can interfere with the way you feel and behave. These factors step up free radical activity in your body and can be detrimental to your health. Look at ways to cut down these risks and improve your quality of living.

RADIATION WAVES

Radio waves, radar, microwaves, televisions, stereos and telephones all contribute to electromagnetic radiation (EMR), which is linked to depression, cataracts, cancers and miscarriage. Look at ways to cut down on exposure to such radiation. Place ionisers wherever there is any kind of electrical equipment and if possible, avoid 'check-up' medical and dental X-rays.

CAFFEINE CONTROL

If your daily intake of caffeine exceeds 350mg (the equivalent of four medium-strength cups of coffee or eight cups of tea), cut down. Otherwise, you can develop irregular breathing, high blood pressure and digestive problems.

SMOKING HAZARDS

Smoking 30 cigarettes a day exposes a smoker to the same degree of radiation as someone who has had 300 chest X-rays in a year. If you give up, ease withdrawal symptoms by taking a high potency B complex supplement (containing at least 50mg each of the major B vitamins such as thiamine and riboflavin) and avoid consuming all stimulant beverages and highly seasoned foods for two to three weeks after you stop smoking.

AIR POLLUTION

Truly clean air has become a rarity. Breathing heavily polluted city air poses similar risks to smoking more than 10 cigarettes a day. Help your body to neutralise inhaled pollutants by taking antioxidant vitamin supplements. If you drive a car, minimise pollution by using lead-free petrol and by having the exhaust system checked regularly. Wear a mask when cycling and avoid jogging near busy roads.

CHEMICAL CONTACT

Swimming in chlorinated water drenches the skin in chemicals. Always shower directly after swimming and smooth on a hydrating body lotion.

BREEDING BACTERIA

Used tea-towels become breeding grounds for bacteria, which can lead to food-borne illnesses. Lower the risks by allowing dishes to dry naturally and wash tea-towels soiled with meat, chicken, fish or milk before reusing them. After handling food, wash your hands with hot water and an antibacterial soap for at least 30 seconds.

FOOD ALERT

Maintaining a healthy diet is not as easy as it sounds. So much of the produce available today is either full of preservatives and additives or contaminated by environmental toxins such as pesticides, industrial dyes and pollutants. All of these can have adverse effects on the body, ranging from allergies to more serious complaints such as skin disorders, digestive ailments and behavioural disorders. To minimise the risks, avoid foods loaded with additives and preservatives and increase your consumption of raw fruit and vegetables. Foods labelled as having 'added vitamins' can be misleading. Manufacturers may be merely replacing the essential nutrients lost during processing.

TOXIC FUMES

Today's synthetic paints are derived mainly from petrochemicals. With concern about the health implications of these chemical compounds on the increase, a safer option is to use paints made from plant oils, tree resins, linseed oil, orange peel oil or canarba wax. Also look for paints that contain natural colour pigments.

WATER SAFETY

Avoid drinking tap water as it is often contaminated by wastes, pesticides and other toxins. It may also carry heavy residues from either copper or lead pipes. Opt for bottled spring water or filtered water.

HEALTHY LIVING

FOLLOW THESE STEPS TO IMPROVE YOUR HEALTH

CLEAR HEAD

To avoid the morning-after effects of excess alcohol consumption, try taking 1000mgs of vitamin C before you go to bed and avoid stimulants such as coffee. In the morning, drink plenty of water and take a B complex vitamin supplement.

PREP WORK _

To maintain the nutritional content of food, always steam, bake, poach or stir-fry. Cook fresh food and avoid reheating meals as this depletes essential nutrients. Steer clear of microwave ovens as the long-term effects of their radiation on the body are unknown.

REGULAR EXERCISE

Step up the activity of your lymphatic system with regular exercise. Lymph is a clear fluid that transports and expels the body's wastes. Poor nutrition and a sedentary lifestyle slow down lymph flow, which causes a build-up of toxins.

JUICING BENEFITS

A one-day juice fast (consuming only fresh fruit and vegetables juices) once a month will cleanse your system. Juices are easy for the body to absorb quickly and efficiently, taking on average only 10–15 minutes to digest.

WAVE LENGTHS

Computer screens carry positive ion charges which attract positive ions from the environment. These ions cause lethargy and tiredness. Use an anti-glare protective screen, sit at least 50cm from your computer and take a break every 20 minutes.

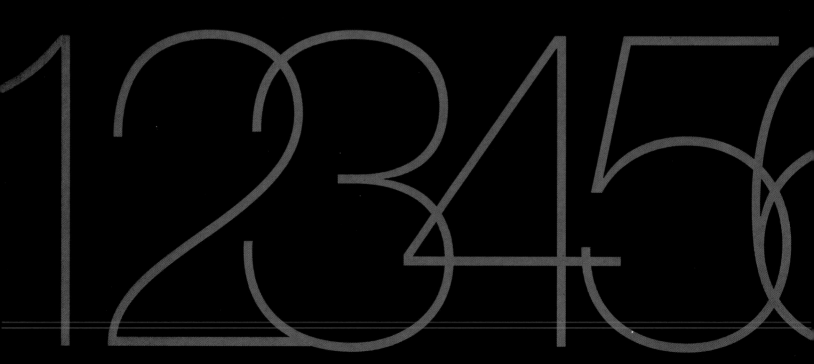

HEALTH CHECKS

Make sure that you have regular medical check-ups and pap smears. Always examine yourself for changes in your body's appearance at home and keep an eye on any changes in moles and suspicious lumps in your breasts.

STRESS EASE

Stress causes chemical reactions in the brain which disrupt the functioning of the organs. An imbalance occurs when your body retains these stresses. To maintain your health, reduce stress by trying different relaxation techniques, such as yoga.

BREATHE DEEPLY

When you're stressed, the adrenal glands go into overdrive. To slow down this activity and induce a state of calm, roll your eyes upwards and then close them. Breathe deeply and slowly count to 10. Concentrate on regulating your breathing.

SUPER GRASS

Wheatgrass juice is a very nutritious drink. Made of almost pure chlorophyll, it contains vital enzymes and vitamins that assist with weight loss and maintain general health. You may feel nauseous after drinking: it's just the juice at work.

TRAVEL EASE

Long-distance travel takes its toll on the body. If you suffer from jetlag, have a bath laced with one drop each of lavender and geranium oil before going to bed, then add two drops of peppermint and eucalyptus oil to your morning bath.

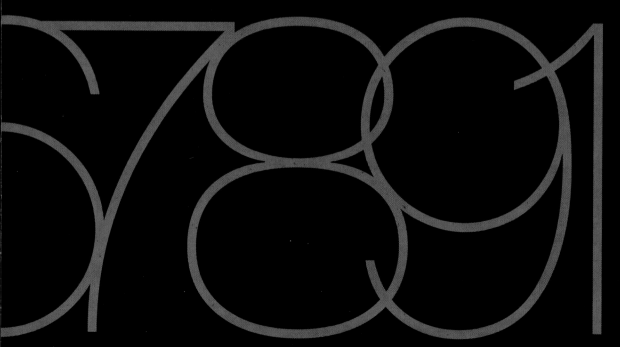
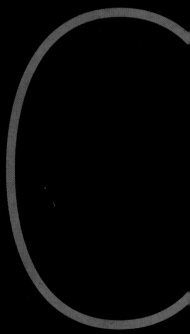

PROBLEM

Do you suffer from hot flushes when the heat is on?

Drinking a cup of hot peppermint tea will have an instantly cooling effect on your system.

Is watching television a good way to induce sleep?

Avoid watching television before going to bed. Rays emitted from television sets can affect your nervous system, which can prevent you from sleeping properly.

What can you do to soothe sunburn?

Add three drops of lavender oil to 600ml cold water. Dip a face-cloth in the solution, wring it out and apply this as a cold compress to the affected area.

How can you calm yourself when you're stressed?

Inhale a whiff of lavender oil, it will have an instant calming effect.

How often should you have an eye test?

To maintain ocular health, the experts recommend that you have your eyes tested once every two years, but more frequently if you have any vision problems.

How can you keep mosquito bites to a minimum?

Eat garlic and foods rich in vitamin B during the summer months to keep the bugs at bay.

Are amalgam fillings in your teeth healthy?

To be on the safe side, have amalgam fillings replaced with porcelain, gold or plastic. Research suggests that amalgam is a potentially toxic material.

Is there a quick fix to ease headaches?

Massage your temples to ease a headache. Lying down with your feet raised on a pillow (so the blood flows back to your head) is also beneficial.

Do you suffer from bad breath?

Taking capsules of peppermint oil after eating neutralises nasty odours. Chewing fennel seeds or parsley will also instantly freshen your breath.

Do you suffer from sore eyes after exposure to harsh weather conditions?

Apply compresses of cool camomile tea bags to your eyelids.

SOLUTION

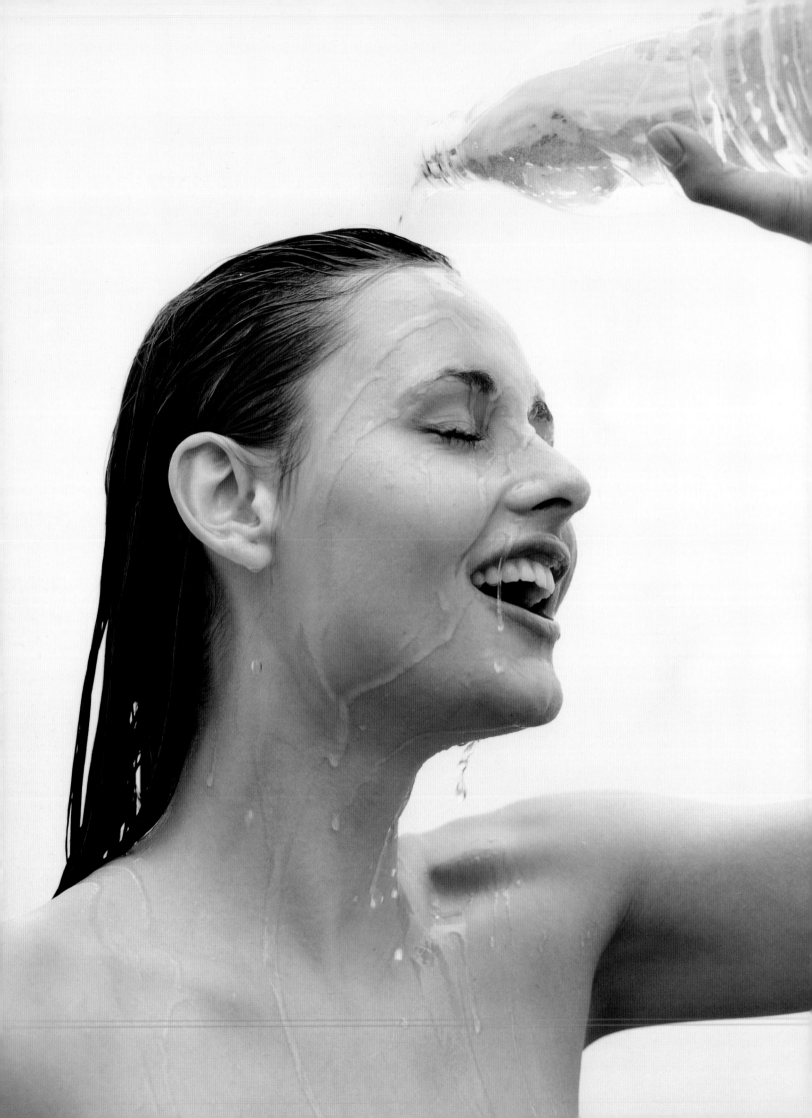

ENERGY

ENERGY IS THE FUEL THAT GIVES YOU DRIVE AND MAINTAINS THE PROPER FUNCTIONING OF YOUR BODY. TO MASTER HIGH-ENERGY LIVING, DE-STRESS SO YOU CAN RE-ENERGISE.

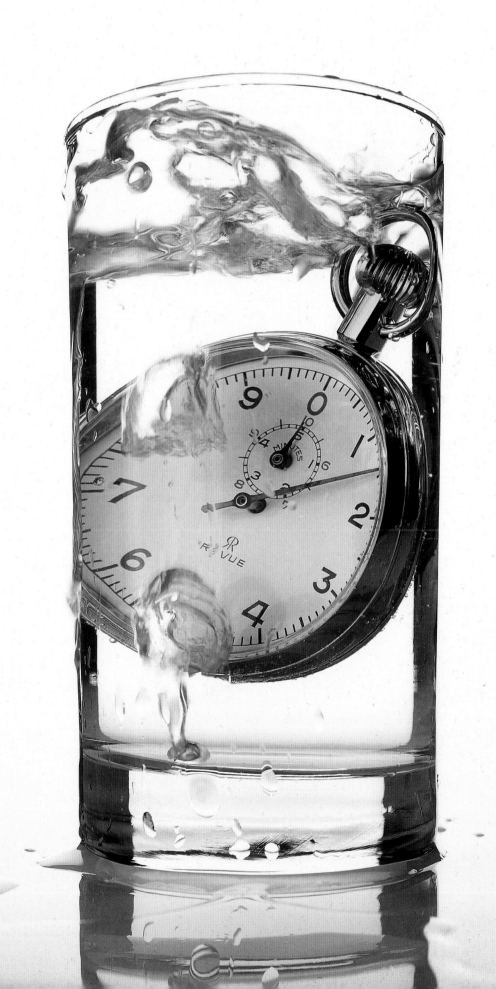

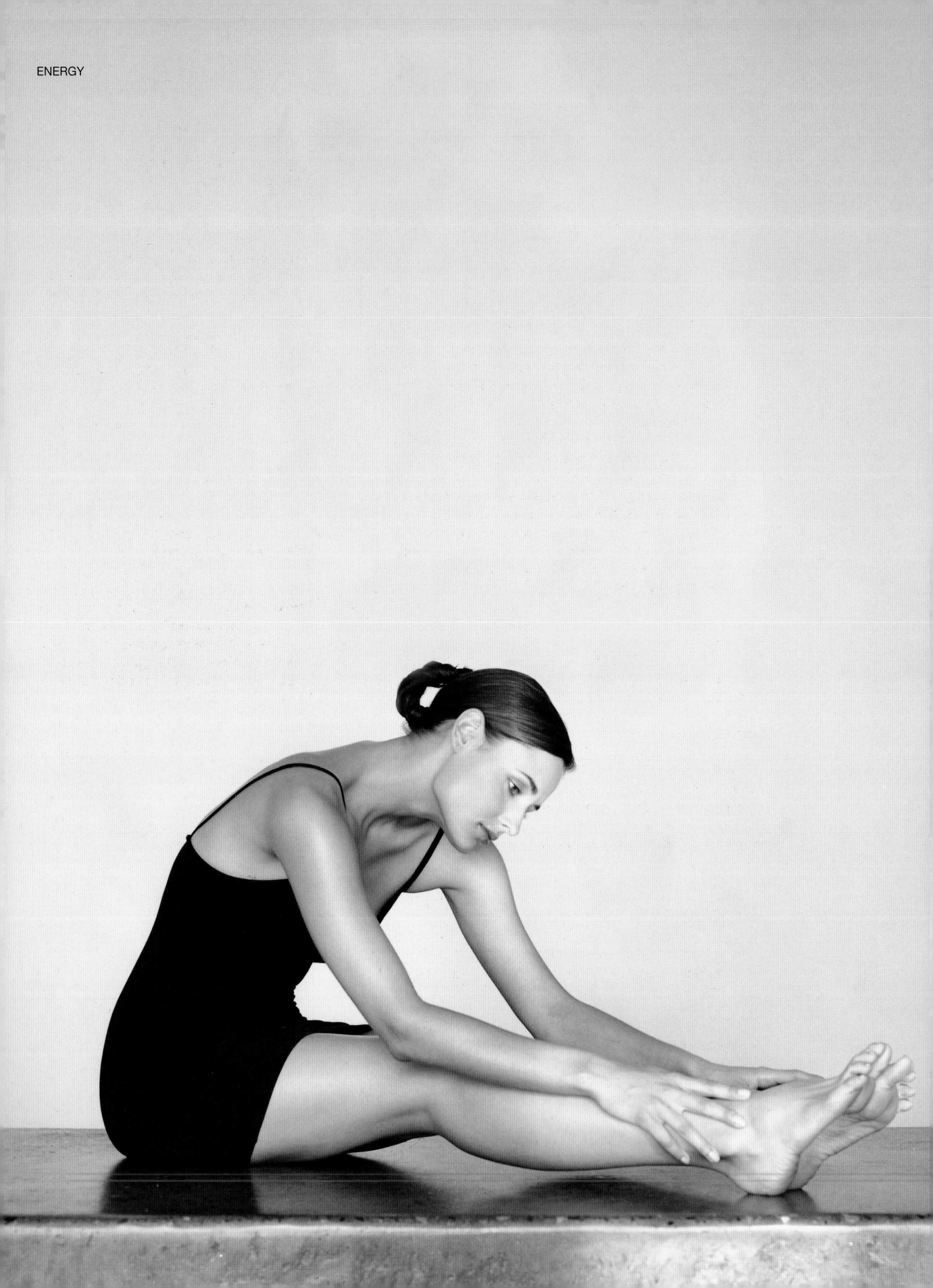

ENERGY FORCE

Do you constantly feel lethargic? Do you need more than eight hours' sleep each night? Are you dependent on a strong cup of coffee to get you going in the morning? Are you too tired to exercise? If any of these apply to you, it's likely that your energy is at a low ebb.

LOW ENERGY LEVELS often indicate that your general health is suffering. Conditions ranging from skin disorders to asthma, premenstrual syndrome (PMS) and high blood pressure are attributed to high stress levels and low energy supplies.

THE TRADITIONS OF ANCIENT ORIENTAL MEDICINE maintain that your energy, known as *chi*, flows through 'meridians' (or pathways) within your body. When these pathways are blocked, energy becomes stuck and imbalances occur, which in turn result in illness and disease. Health and well-being are restored when the energy is flowing freely again.

ENERGY SAPPERS

Stress is a major contributory factor in the depletion of energy resources. Other energy sappers include lack of exercise, over-consumption of sugar and processed foods, and external factors such as noise pollution and chemicals.

THERE IS A COMPLEX CHAIN OF CHEMICAL REACTIONS within your cells that is controlled by the body's supply of vitamins and minerals. When supplies of these substances are low, energy production suffers. If you are aware of these potential energy sappers, you can eliminate them from your lifestyle, or at least learn to deal with them so that they no longer have a harmful effect on your body.

STRESS MANAGEMENT

When you experience stress, your body reacts by releasing adrenaline, a hormone that causes your blood pressure to rise and your heart rate to increase. Adrenaline also stimulates the release of fatty acids and glucose (the body's main energy supplier) into the bloodstream. When you are stressed for prolonged periods, the changes in levels of circulating fats and blood within your body may cause dizziness, weakness and a lack of energy. The symptoms of stress include an inability to concentrate, anxiety, irritability and lethargy.

WHEN YOU HAVE MUSCULAR TENSION, a large amount of your energy is wasted. Under normal conditions, your muscles use more energy than any other part of the body and this increases when you're feeling stressed.

ENERGY BOOSTS

A whiff of peppermint oil will have an energising effect on the mind and body. Add a few drops to a tissue or cotton handkerchief and when you're feeling tired, deeply inhale the aroma.

Avoid stressful situations, they deplete vital energy reserves. Make changes in your lifestyle to lower levels of stress. For example, if travelling to work during peak hour rattles you, leave earlier or later to avoid the traffic.

Have a protein boost. Lean proteins such as fish and chicken contain iron, which increases the production of red blood cells. Iron also contains B vitamins, which help to increase energy levels.

Raw juices cleanse the body by shifting unwanted toxins. This in turn gives you more energy. Try following a fresh fruit and raw vegetable detoxing regime. For a cleansing cup, opt for celery, spinach and apple juices and for an energising drink, try a blend of carrot and soy milk.

STRESS RELIEF
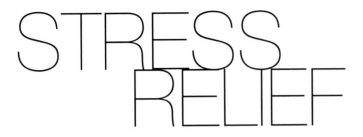

Stress tolerance levels differ among individuals, but with regular exercise, massage and different relaxation techniques, you can maintain effective stress management.

NUTRITION

Since your body loses its reserves of vitamins B and C and zinc rapidly when the pressure is on, good nutrition is an effective way to deal with stress. Step up your intake of green vegetables, fresh fruit, wholegrain cereals, nuts, seeds and dried fruit to replace vitamin B (which boosts your immune system); citrus fruits, (especially kiwi fruit) to replace vitamin C; and liver, dairy produce, red meat and shellfish for zinc (both vitamin C and zinc are essential in the fight against infection).

SOOTHING SOUNDS

Sound therapy can have a powerful effect on your health. It is reputed to reduce stress, lower blood pressure, alleviate pain and even help to overcome learning disabilities. Harmonious tunes prompt the brain to emit a hormone known as ACTH (adrenocorticotrophic hormone). ACTH helps to control the production of adrenaline (which is released in large amounts into the bloodstream when under stress) and has a calming effect on the brain. Music also triggers the release of endorphins, the body's natural feel-good chemicals. To calm fraught nerves and reduce tension, relax and tune into some soothing sounds.

YOGA

Yoga is an ancient practice that combines relaxation and exercise for both mind and body. It is an ideal way to reduce stress levels and to restore the natural equilibrium of your body. There are different types of yoga techniques. The safest way to practise yoga is to work with a professional instructor to begin with.

MEDITATION

To ease stress, try meditation. Either consult the experts to learn professionally or use this simple technique: find a quiet spot and sit with your legs crossed, back straight and palms facing up, resting on your knees. Close your eyes and completely relax. Inhale deeply through your nose and exhale through your mouth. Repeat this several times and either focus your thoughts on an object or imagine white light. Remain in this relaxed state for at least 15 minutes.

FLOATATION TANKS

Floatation tanks are the perfect place in which to relax and unwind. You lie on your back in 25–30cm of salty, buoyant water in a small, dark, enclosed chamber, listening to soothing music. The floatation has a calming effect on your mind, body and spirit and will reduce levels of stress-related biochemicals within your body. Floatation tanks are not recommended if you suffer from claustrophobia.

SLEEP TIGHT

Difficulty sleeping or waking up in the morning feeling anxious are indicators that you are suffering from stress. To ensure a successful night's sleep, dab a couple of drops of lavender oil onto your pillow before going to bed. Alternatively, soak a pair of cotton socks in cold water, wring them out and put them on your feet. Then place a dry pair of socks over the top. The cold sensation will instantly draw energy down to your feet and you'll feel calm and relaxed.

Although you shouldn't go to bed with a full stomach, there are certain foods that may actually help you to sleep. Try snacking on bananas, figs, dates, yoghurt or wholegrain crackers. Drink a glass of warm milk before going to bed, as it contains tryptophan, a precursor of one of the brain's calming chemicals.

If you decide to take sleeping tablets, opt for a natural version. Passionflower, hop and valerian root are all plant remedies that instil a sense of calm without any of the adverse side effects commonly associated with chemical tranquillisers. These are available from health food stores.

AROMATHERAPY

A bath infused with aromatherapy oils can ease stress and tension. Try lacing warm water with six drops of lavender or camomile oil and wallow in the tub for 10 minutes. Alternatively, soak a face-cloth in warm water and three drops of lavender oil, and then wring it out. Lie down, put your feet up (rest them on a pillow) and place this compress on your fore-head for 10 minutes.

SHIATSU MASSAGE

If you're stressed, a professional shiatsu massage will ease tension. The Japanese interpretation of Chinese acupuncture, shiatsu, (meaning 'finger pressure'), involves the exertion of firm pressure on different points of the body that relate to different organs and energy path-ways. This addresses imbalances and ensures that the body's energy, which often becomes sluggish and blocked due to stress, flows freely. Shiatsu is an invigorating massage, rather than a relaxing experience.

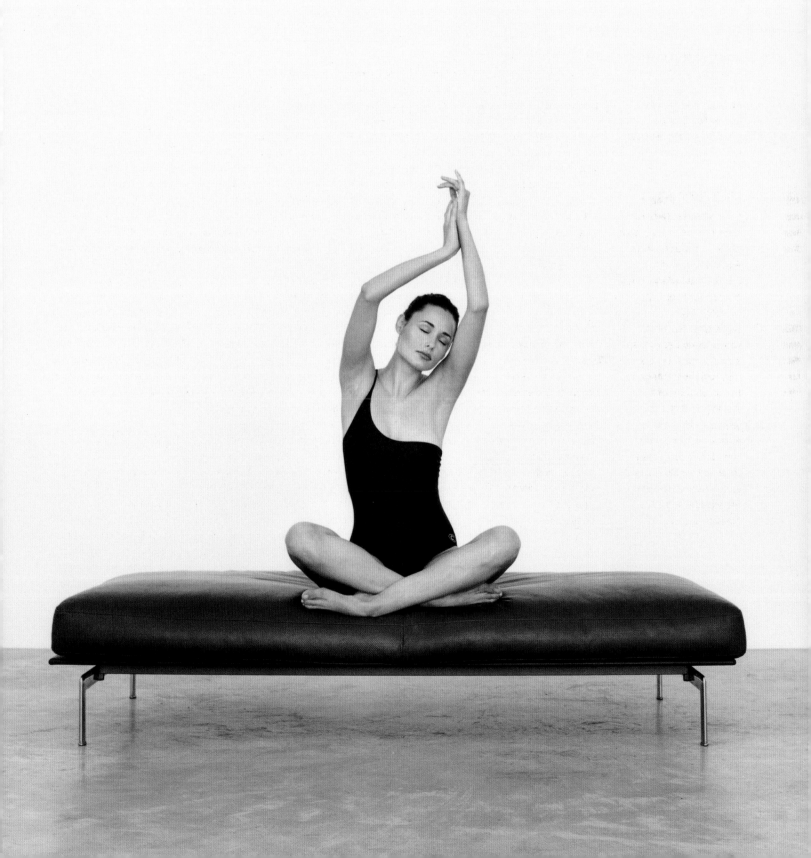

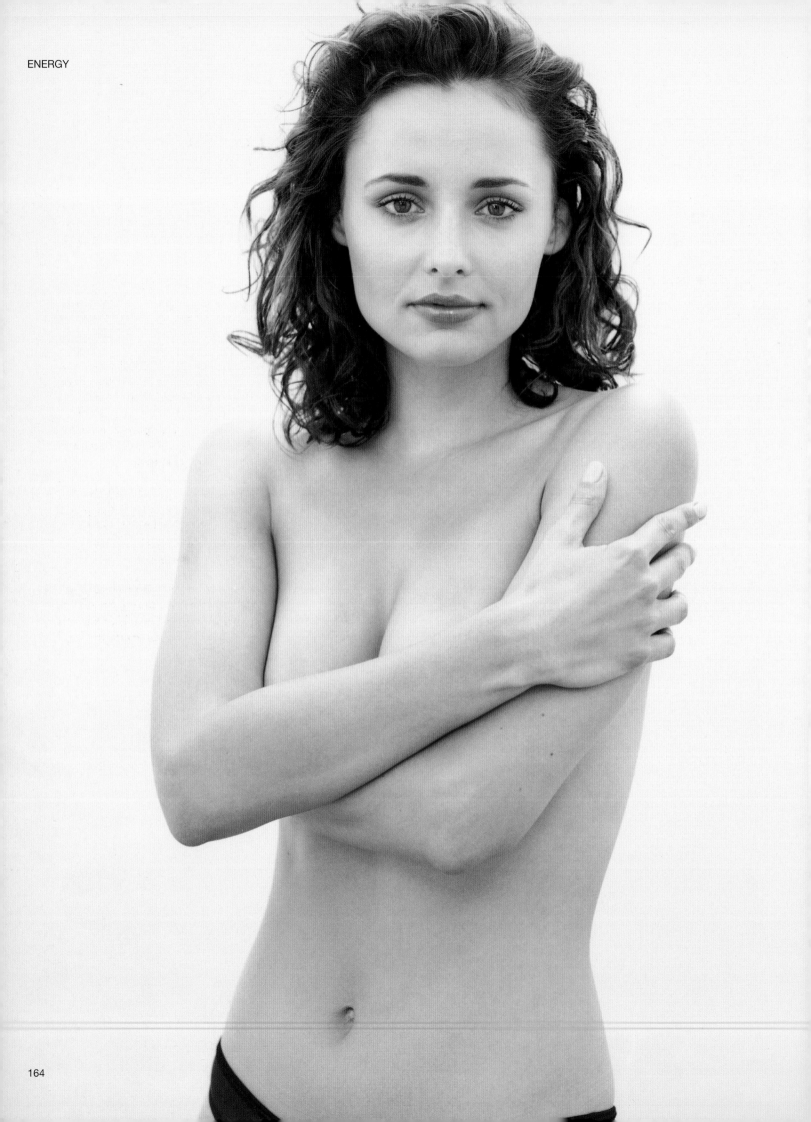

HIGH-ENERGY LIVING

Making simple changes to your lifestyle can have a noticeable effect on your energy levels and can also play a vital role in stress management. Once you've broken bad habits and locked into a positive cycle, you will notice a dramatic improvement in the way you feel.

EXERCISE

Any form of physical activity will increase your energy levels and improve your overall health. Exercise triggers the release of natural, pleasure-enhancing chemicals in the brain known as endorphins, which produce the 'natural high' felt during physical activity. Try to include 25–30 minutes of aerobic exercise such as walking, running, dancing or cycling into your regime three times a week to maximise energy levels.

IF YOU EAT MORE FOOD THAN YOUR BODY BURNS in energy, the surplus is stored as fat. Regular exercise will help keep your body in shape and fat deposits under control.

COLONIC IRRIGATION

Stress, poor diet and drugs all inhibit the functioning of the colon and block it with toxic waste. These toxins are released into the bloodstream and have a negative impact on your health. If you feel sluggish, tired or your general health is suffering, colonic irrigation can be beneficial. In a typical irrigation session, an applicator, or speculum, is inserted into the anus and several litres of water are flushed around the colon, dislodging and flushing out toxins. Taking the poisons out of your body will boost energy levels and restore health.

COLOUR THERAPY

Research confirms that specific colours have a psychological effect on both mind and body. Red is reputed to excite the body, and increase the heart rate, brain activity and respiration. Blue has the opposite effect, making it ideal as a relaxant. Yellow lifts the spirits, stimulates the memory and increases the pulse rate. Purple induces feelings of liberation. When you're in need of an energy fix, focus on an object or a piece of paper of your chosen colour for several minutes. Your subconscious mind will respond and send out signals to the rest of your body to address its needs.

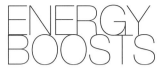

ENERGY BOOSTS

Give up smoking. Apart from the well-known serious health effects, nicotine robs the vitamins and minerals essential for energy production.

Limit your alcohol intake as excess amounts can interfere with your sleeping patterns, which in turn affects your well-being.

Reflexology sessions can boost energy levels. This ancient practice focuses on exerting pressure on specific points located on the feet that relate to specific body parts. This treatment readdresses the body's energy flow, relieves stress and is beneficial for general health.

Eat foods rich in vitamin B, such as fruit and vegetables, wheatgerm, seeds, nuts, whole grains, fish and dairy produce. Vitamin B is required for the production of energy.

Eating large meals in one sitting can leave you feeling drained afterwards. To prevent this from happening, the experts recommend eating small meals often.

EATING FOR ENERGY

The foods you eat are converted by your body into glucose and burned as energy. Although fat and, to a lesser extent, protein supply fuel for the body, carbohydrates are the best-known foods to provide physical energy.

CARBOHYDRATES, the starches and sugars found in fruits, vegetables, cereals and grains, are broken down gradually by your body and release sugar slowly into the bloodstream, providing a long-lasting source of energy.

THE BODY ABSORBS DIFFERENT CARBOHYDRATES at different rates. For an instant energy boost, snack on bananas, dates, raisins, dried apricots, rice, wholemeal bread or wholegrain cereals. For a longer-lasting, steadier energy supply, eat complex carbohydrates such as baked beans, lentils, porridge oats, pasta, potatoes, apples, oatmeal biscuits or muesli.

FAST FIXES

The key to maintaining energy supplies is to keep your blood sugar level constant. Hypoglycaemia (low blood sugar) is the reason you can feel full of life one minute and drained the next. To prevent your energy levels from fluctuating, avoid stimulants such as coffee or chocolate and sugary or refined foods. They offer a fast energy fix by sending blood sugar levels soaring, but energy levels drop soon afterwards. If you have a sugar craving, the natural sugars found in fruit provide energy, as well as other valuable vitamins and minerals. This type of sugar fix offers a longer-term energy release, so you won't experience feelings of lethargy shortly after you eat.

SUGAR OVERLOAD

A diet containing too much refined sugar can lead to glucose intolerance. This is when the body is unable to maintain blood sugar levels, resulting in fatigue, dizziness, depression, digestive problems, insomnia and excess thirst. If you suffer from this condition, stay away from coffee, chocolate, sugar, refined foods, cigarettes, alcohol and increase your consumption of complex carbohydrates.

ENERGY ESSENCE

During its complex energy production process, your body facilitates the production of serotonin, a hormone that creates feelings of satisfaction and relaxation. If your body doesn't maintain optimum energy levels, your brain won't receive relaxing signals from serotonin. This leads to constant hunger pangs and, potentially, unnecessary weight gain.

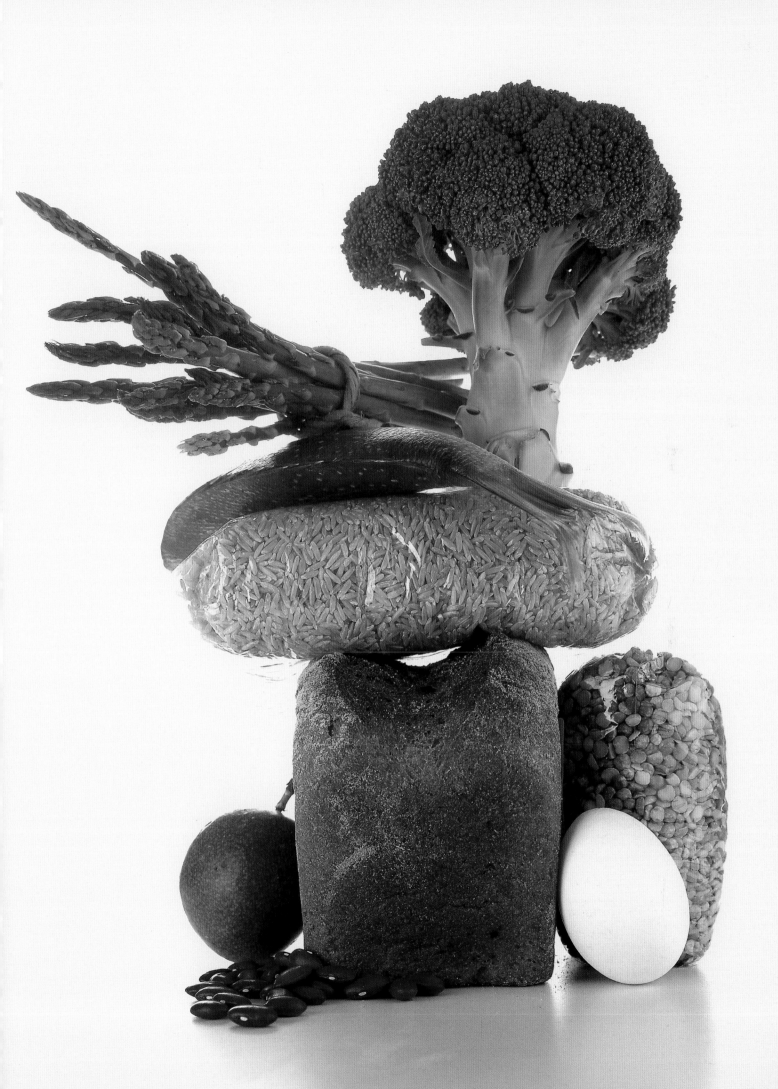

ENERGY BOOSTS

FOLLOW THESE STEPS TO REVITALISE YOURSELF

GARLIC FIX

Eat a clove of garlic every day. Garlic is a rich source of germanium, a mineral that has proved to be valuable in the improvement of energy production cycles. Garlic also contains over 10 antioxidants, which help to slow down the ageing process.

OILY BENEFITS

Incorporate two or three tablespoons of cold-pressed flaxseed oil into your daily diet. Mix it with yoghurt or use it as a dressing on salads. Flaxseed oil ensures the body is supplied with sufficient essential fatty acids, which are needed to produce energy and sustain general health.

BREATHE DEEPLY

As you breathe, you unconsciously release tension and boost energy, but shallow breathing doesn't achieve this effect. For maximum impact, try taking deep breaths down into your abdomen, then exhale and relax. Repeat until you feel refreshed.

ENERGY POINT

Exerting pressure on specific body zones boosts energy. Find the pressure point in the web of your thumb and forefinger. Pinch this point firmly with the thumb and forefinger of your other hand. Hold this for a maximum of two minutes and then release gradually.

BANANA BOOST

A banana is a far better source of energy than a bar of chocolate. The humble banana's high concentration of natural sugar produces a slow, long-lasting energy boost, whereas the quick sugar fix from chocolate gives you an instant high followed by a sharp drop in energy.

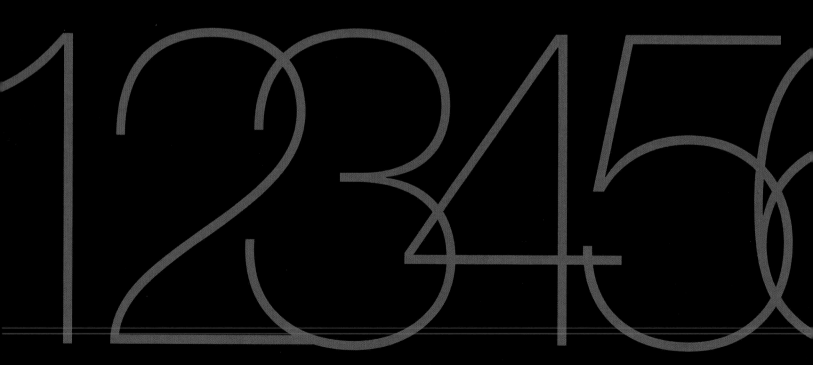

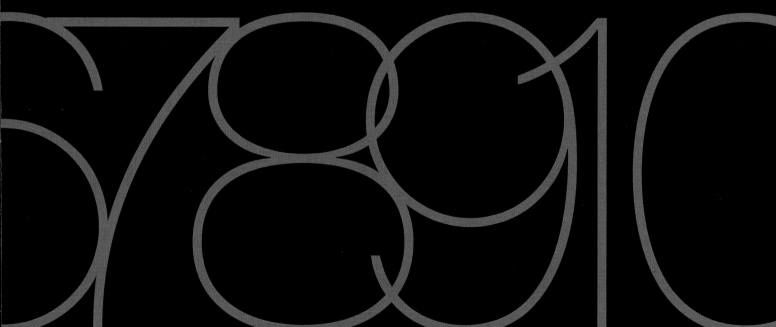

PACE WORK

A brisk walk works wonders when you're feeling tired as it stimulates the heart, lungs, muscles and mind. Walking for at least 30 minutes three times a week will boost energy levels and help to burn unwanted fat, as long as you walk at a moderate to brisk pace.

JUST JUICE

When your energy levels are low, concoct your own drink to provide you with all the energy you need. Mix one banana, one mango, half a medium-sized pineapple, 150ml milk or a small carton of plain, low-fat yoghurt and one teaspoon of honey in a blender.

NATURAL HABITS

Keep your natural body rhythms consistent. Aim to go to bed and wake at the same time each day whenever possible. Also, your nutritional habits significantly affect energy levels: the experts recommend eating small meals often and only snacking on nutritious food.

FLEXING BOOST

If you're feeling tired, try this simple stretch to give yourself an instant boost: stand up straight with your feet apart. Slowly raise your arms above your head, inhaling deeply. Hold for 10 seconds and then exhale as you lower your arms. Repeat until you feel refreshed.

GREEN FRIENDS

Radiation from video players, TVs and computers can interfere with hormonal balances and cause lethargy. Surround yourself with green plants. They break down radiation and produce supplies of oxygen, ideal if you work in an aircond-itioned environment.

MASSAGE

Whether you opt for professional or DIY home treatment, massage can be a powerful experience that conditions the mind, body and spirit. Massage stimulates lymphatic drainage to shift unwanted toxins from the body – helping to relieve stress, to soothe aching muscles, to release emotional tension and to pep up circulation. Lymph is a clear fluid that flows around the body, transporting toxins to waste disposal sites. Massage movements stimulate muscle contractions, which in turn promotes lymphatic flow.

TOUCH STROKES

Massage strokes should work in harmony with blood flow: always toward the heart. Different massage strokes benefit different parts of the body.

EFFLEURAGE involves light, flowing strokes that warm and relax the muscles and boost lymph flow. Use your whole hand, and always start and finish a massage with these strokes.

PETRISSAGE is a kneading motion that involves the exertion of firm pressure (without causing pain). Literally squeeze and roll the flesh between your thumb and fingers. These movements are beneficial for fatty areas of the body, such as the thighs.

TAPOTEMENT, also known as percussion, refers to flicking, cupping and chopping motions using the hands. The wrists should be loose and flexible and the movements fast and invigorating. *Tapotement* improves muscle and skin tone and is ideal for relieving tension in the back and pummelling fatty areas on the backs of the legs.

FRICTION is a rapid oscillating movement that soothes stiff joints and promotes blood flow. Using your fingers and thumbs, focus deeply on smaller areas of the body in rhythmic movements.

MASSAGE OILS

Moisturiser can be used as a massage aid, but oil is more beneficial as it enables the hands to glide easily over the body. Use sweet almond, avocado, jojoba or apricot oil and for extra therapeutic benefits, blend one of these base oils with your favourite essential oil.

EXPERT ADVICE

For a relaxing massage oil, blend four drops of lavender oil, four drops of patchouli oil, two drops of rose oil and 20ml sweet almond oil.

For an invigorating blend, mix three drops each of bergamot, grapefruit and rosemary oil with 20ml base oil such as avocado or apricot kernel oil.

Avoid stimulants such as coffee, nicotine and alcohol before a massage.

For a head massage, apply your favourite essential oil (diluted in a base oil) to your fingertips and over your scalp. Splay your fingers out and gently knead your scalp, working from the front of your head down to the nape of your neck.

After an aerobic workout, work over the body with *petrissage* movements when you're in the shower to release toxins and prevent muscular aches.

To ease period pain, apply spot pressure to the acupressure points located just behind the tips of the ankle bones. Hold firmly for 10–15 seconds.

Wheatgerm oil is rich in vitamin E, which makes it ideal for massage if you have post-operative scars or stretch marks.

Lymphatic drainage massage is the perfect treatment if you're feeling sluggish or tired. This type of massage shifts unwanted toxins, regulates lymph flow and boosts energy levels.

SELF-MASSAGE

Get to grips with massage and give yourself a top-to-toe treat with the following 10-minute program. If you want a longer massage, repeat each movement several times.

ARMS & HANDS

Smooth oil over your hands and up your arms in sweeping motions. Repeat five times. Squeeze each forearm between the fingers and heel of the other hand. Work along the upper arm, concentrating on the centre muscles and use *petrissage* movements on the underside. Massage your hands, kneading the palms, then grasp each finger between your thumb and forefinger and gently pull from the joint to the fingertip.

NECK & SHOULDERS

Warm oil in your palms and smooth it onto your neck and shoulders. Press and rotate the fingers of each hand into the muscles at the base of your neck (on either side of the vertebrae) up to the base of your skull. Work to the sides of your neck and repeat, alternating between firm and gentle pressure. Work over your shoulders with firm *petrissage* strokes using your fingers and palms. Work back and forth from the shoulder to the neck. Squeeze the shoulder muscles between the fingers and heel of your hand to relieve tension.

TORSO & ABDOMEN

Apply oil across the upper half of your chest in sweeping motions. Work from your shoulders down to the pectoral chest muscles (avoiding breast tissue) and gently squeeze between the fingers and heel of your hand, one side at a time. Then lie down and smooth oil over your abdomen. Massage in circular movements in a clockwise direction only (to follow the direction of the colon and stimulate digestion). This can relieve a bloated stomach. Use *petrissage* and gently knead the flesh on your stomach and around the centre of your body.

LEGS

After smoothing on oil, use *effleurage* to stroke up each leg five times. Sit down and work over each calf, squeezing the muscles between the thumb and fingers, using both hands. Move up to your thighs. Push the knuckles into the thigh region and use *tapotement* movements. Finish with sweeping motions.

FEET

Massage oil over each foot with *effleurage* movements. Knead the soles using your thumbs, working in firm, circular motions. Then work on the upper feet: press and glide the thumbs between the bones on the top of the feet. Squeeze each toe.

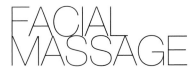

FACIAL MASSAGE

Localised massage relaxes facial muscles, improves circulation and revives the complexion. With these simple steps you can incorporate a three- to five-minute massage into your existing beauty regime at night or, for a longer facial treat, repeat each movement several times. For the maximum benefit, when applying pressure to specific points, hold for 30 seconds.

Forehead Massage upwards from the centre of your forehead and slide fingers along the hairline. Finish with gentle pressure at the temples. Repeat three times.

Eyes Gently massage around your eyes and over your eyelids with light, tapping motions. Press the point located between the eyes with your middle fingers. Finish by lightly pressing both temples.

Cheeks Glide your hands over your cheekbones, working inward around the delicate eye area. Apply pressure as you work along the contour of the cheekbone. (This will stimulate the colon and the kidneys.) Finish by sweeping your hands down your nose and across the lower region of your cheeks.

Nose & mouth Stroke both sides of your nose with your fingertips, pressing around your nostrils to stimulate circulation. Then follow the contour of your lips, gliding your hands towards the outer corners of the upper lip. Press the central point on the upper lip (below your nose) to encourage the proper functioning of your liver and lymphatic system. Work under the lower lip, massaging upwards, lifting and encircling your mouth.

Chin & neck Using your middle and index fingers, massage your chin, working towards the ear. Repeat three times, then work your hands down your neck using *petrissage* movements.

Ears Massage your ears by starting on the ear lobes. Grab them with your thumb and index finger and gently pull them, stroking them in the process. Repeat this motion, working along the ear.

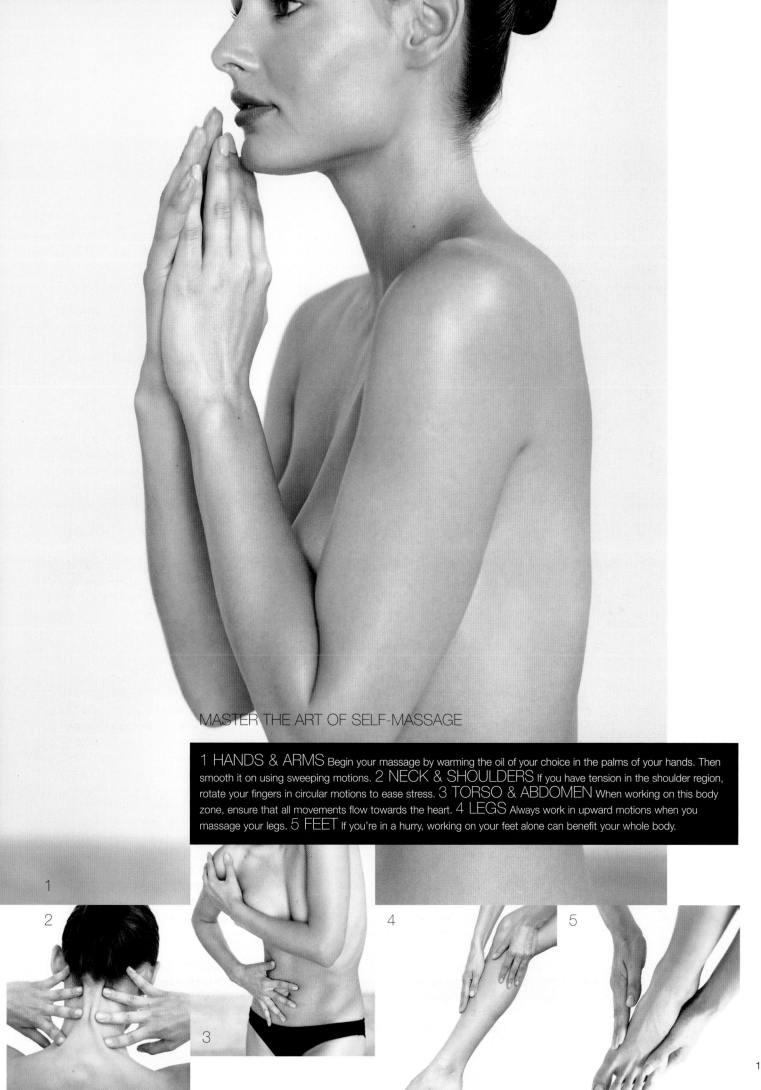

MASTER THE ART OF SELF-MASSAGE

1 HANDS & ARMS Begin your massage by warming the oil of your choice in the palms of your hands. Then smooth it on using sweeping motions. 2 NECK & SHOULDERS If you have tension in the shoulder region, rotate your fingers in circular motions to ease stress. 3 TORSO & ABDOMEN When working on this body zone, ensure that all movements flow towards the heart. 4 LEGS Always work in upward motions when you massage your legs. 5 FEET If you're in a hurry, working on your feet alone can benefit your whole body.

1

2

3

4

5

AROMA POWER

Aromatherapy is an ancient tradition that uses oils extracted from plants and flowers to treat the mind, body and spirit. These oils enter the bloodstream via the skin within 20–70 minutes of application and are reputed to continue working for up to 12 hours. They also stimulate receptors in the nose which relay messages to the limbic system (the part of the brain that regulates the emotions).

NEVER APPLY NEAT ESSENTIAL OILS directly to your skin (lavender and tea-tree oil are the only exceptions), as they are too strong and can burn the skin or cause allergic reactions. Always dilute essential oils with base (or carrier) oils such as sweet almond, jojoba or apricot kernel oil.

AROMATHERAPY TREATS

The benefits of aromatic oils can be incorporated into daily life. Massage is the most effective means of application as the essential oils enter the bloodstream at such a rapid rate. In addition to the aromatic benefits, massage strokes pep up circulation and ease tension.

AROMATIC BATHS can be relaxing or invigorating, depending on your choice of oils. For the maximum impact, add four to eight drops of your favourite essential oil to the bath once the water has run (if you add oils to running water the vapours will evaporate too quickly). Agitate the water to disperse the oil droplets and then immerse yourself in the tub, relax and inhale for at least 10 minutes.

COMPRESSES help treat muscular aches and pains, reduce swelling and bruising, and generally decongest the body. Cold compresses are particularly effective for sports injuries. Add six drops of essential oil to a bowl of 500ml icy cold water. Place a towel or face-cloth into the bowl, leave it to soak, wring it out and apply it to the body. Leave the compress on until it warms to body temperature or dries out. Hot compresses are ideal for backache, rheumatic and arthritic pain, earache and toothache. Follow the above guidelines, but use hot water instead of cold. Place the compress on the affected area, then bind it in cling wrap to retain the heat. Leave the compress on until it cools.

INHALATIONS can relieve colds, flu and sinusitis, revive flagging spirits and boost energy levels. Add one drop each of tea-tree and peppermint oil to a bowl of near-boiling water. Place your head over the bowl, drape a towel over your head and the bowl and breathe in the vapours for five minutes.

VAPORISING OILS in a burner can influence your mood, create a relaxing ambience and disguise nasty cooking aromas or cigarette smoke. Burn six drops of your favourite essential oil and a small amount of water in an oil burner.

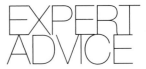

EXPERT ADVICE

Consult an aromatherapist before using essential oils if you are pregnant (the essences can affect the foetus), if you suffer from an illness such as epilepsy, or if you have a heart condition.

Citrus oils, especially bergamot oil, increase the skin's sensitivity to sunlight. Avoid using these oils during exposure to ultraviolet light.

Skin sensitivity and allergies can be aggravated by essential oils. Always do a skin patch test with an essential oil (diluted in a base oil) before using it, or consult an aromatherapist.

Avoid showering, bathing or drinking alcohol after an aromatic massage, as the oils work for up to 12 hours after they are applied.

Essential oils are guaranteed to last for up to 12 months, depending on the type of oil. For example, citrus oils only last six months, and neroli lasts for 12 months.

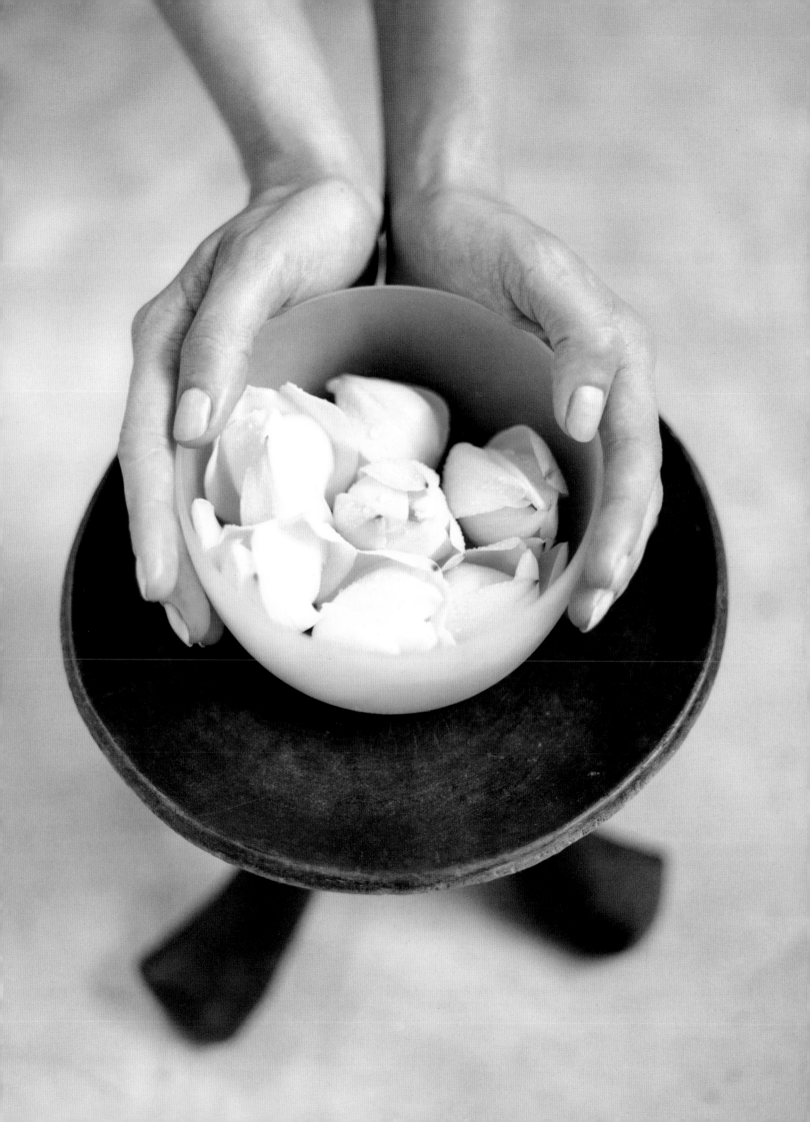

ESSENTIAL OILS

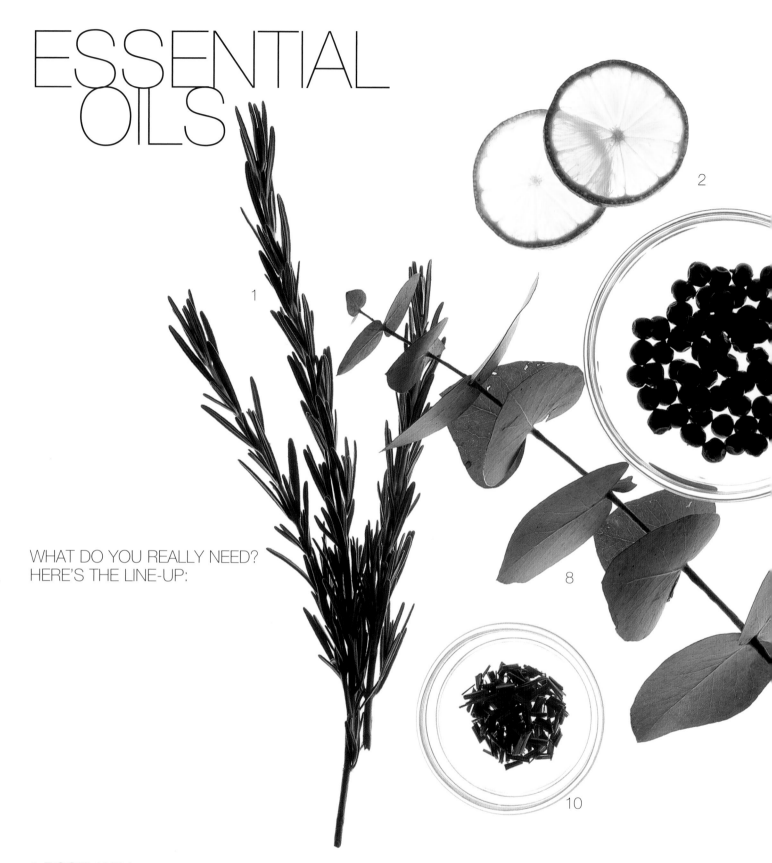

WHAT DO YOU REALLY NEED?
HERE'S THE LINE-UP:

1 ROSEMARY enhances mental clarity and treats rheumatic problems, oily hair, dandruff, headaches, exhaustion and stress. Blend it with lavender and frankincense to reinforce the anti-rheumatic properties. 2 LEMON has an invigorating aroma and helps with circulatory complaints, oily skin, acne, boils, chilblains, high blood pressure, sore throats, colds and catarrh. 3 GERANIUM is good for poor circulation and PMS. It balances hormones, mood swings and depression. 4 LEMON VERBENA is used for its calming properties. 5 JUNIPER has antiseptic properties that benefit oily skin and scalp, colds, arthritis and rheumatic complaints, and muscular aches and pains. It blends well with bergamot, lavender, neroli, rosemary and sandalwood. 6 CINNAMON can be burnt as an anti-depressant as it has a rich, warm and uplifting aroma. It blends well with citrus,

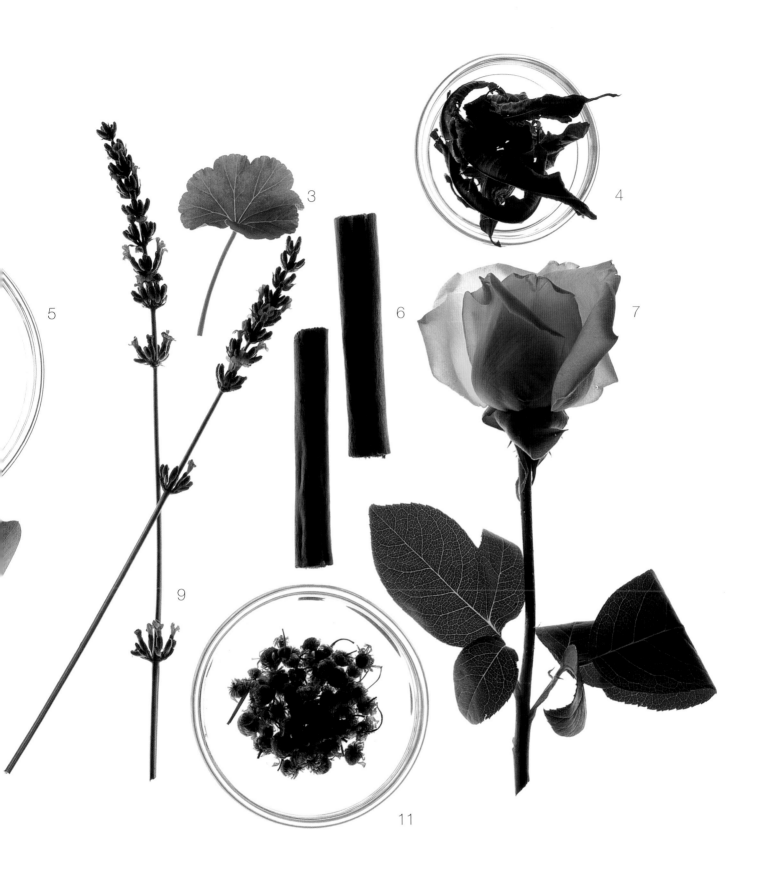

3

4

5

6

7

9

11

clove, ginger and frankincense oils. 7 ROSE has anti-inflammatory and antiseptic properties and benefits dry skins, thread veins, nausea, depression, insomnia and PMS. 8 EUCALYPTUS has antiseptic, stimulating and deodorising effects. It treats burns, blisters, muscular aches and pains, poor circulation and helps to keep insects at bay. 9 LAVENDER is known for its ability to soothe and heal. It is suitable for treating acne, allergies, tinea, insect bites and stings, headaches, insomnia and stress-related disorders. 10 LEMON GRASS smells sweet and has an earthy undertone. It treats tinea, muscular aches and pains, bad circulation, fever, infections, nervous exhaustion and stress. 11 CAMOMILE has a calming effect and is beneficial for inflamed skin, insomnia and PMS. It blends well with citrus oils, lavender, geranium, jasmine, neroli, rose and ylang ylang oils.

AROMATIC REMEDIES

Use essential oils to treat health and beauty problems (unless you are pregnant). Create the following aromatherapy blends to treat different ailments. You can also use them as massage preparations or as therapeutic bath remedies.

PROBLEM SKIN

Treat acne or greasy skin with a blend of five drops of cypress, 10 drops of lemon and five drops of petitgrain oil added to 50ml base oil to balance the condition. To zap the odd blemish, apply neat lavender or tea-tree oil to the affected area using a cotton bud.

DRY AND NORMAL SKIN

Dry and normal skin types will benefit from a blend of five drops of geranium, four drops of jasmine and 16 drops of lavender in 50ml base oil. Massage this blend into freshly cleansed skin at night.

PREMENSTRUAL SYNDROME (PMS)

Forty per cent of women suffer from PMS. Create a blend to suit your needs and add it to your bath or use it as a body oil. For the best results, massage the oil over your abdomen, hips and lower back, focusing on the coccyx (the lower end of the backbone). For bathing, concoct your blend and then add seven to nine drops once the water has run. If you feel irritable, try blending five drops of lavender, five drops of geranium, 10 drops of bergamot with 30ml base oil. If you feel tired and lifeless, mix six drops of grapefruit, six drops of mandarin or orange and two drops of basil with 30ml base oil. If you feel emotional, use a blend of four drops of neroli, five drops of bergamot and five drops of lavender with 30ml base oil.

PSORIASIS

Mix one drop each of bergamot and lavender oil with 5ml sweet almond oil. Massage into problem areas.

FLU

If you feel the symptoms of flu coming on, have a warm bath laced with five drops of tea-tree oil, two drops of lavender and two drops of thyme. Afterwards, pat your skin dry with a towel. Next massage your body with two drops of tea-tree oil and three drops of eucalyptus oil mixed with a teaspoon of almond oil. Go straight to bed.

MUSCLE STRAINS

To soothe tired, aching muscles, apply a cold compress. Add 10 drops of camomile, lavender or rosemary oil to a bowl of cold water. Soak a face-cloth in the preparation, wring it out and place it on the aching area. Leave it on until it warms to body temperature or dries out.

FAINTING

Put a couple of drops of marjoram and lavender oils onto a tissue and hold it under the nose of someone who has fainted to revive them.

ANXIETY

Problems including stress, anxiety and tension, which are associated with the nervous system, will benefit from a balancing blend of five drops of clary sage, five drops of lemon and five drops of lavender in 30ml base oil. Use this blend as a body rub, bath preparation or in a burner in your workplace.

SLUGGISH CIRCULATION

Sluggish circulation can be the result of cold weather, lack of exercise, or an unhealthy diet. Blend four drops each of lemon, juniper, grapefruit and geranium oil with 30ml base oil and use it as a massage preparation. Use invigorating massage strokes to help step up the body's blood flow.

SWOLLEN ANKLES

Swelling can result from high blood pressure, varicose veins, water retention or by standing for prolonged periods. To treat this condition, try an invigorating foot bath. Fill a bowl with warm water and add one drop each of cypress and lavender oil. Soak your feet in the bath for 10 minutes.

ECZEMA

Treat eczema with a topical application made from two drops each of bergamot, lavender and camomile oil mixed with two teaspoons of almond oil. To soothe itchy skin, mix four drops of lavender oil in two teaspoons of cider vinegar and smooth it onto the affected area. Alternatively, try applying a lukewarm aromatic compress to the affected skin. Blend one drop of camomile oil in warm water, soak a face-cloth in the preparation, wring it out and then place it on the patch of eczema for 10 minutes.

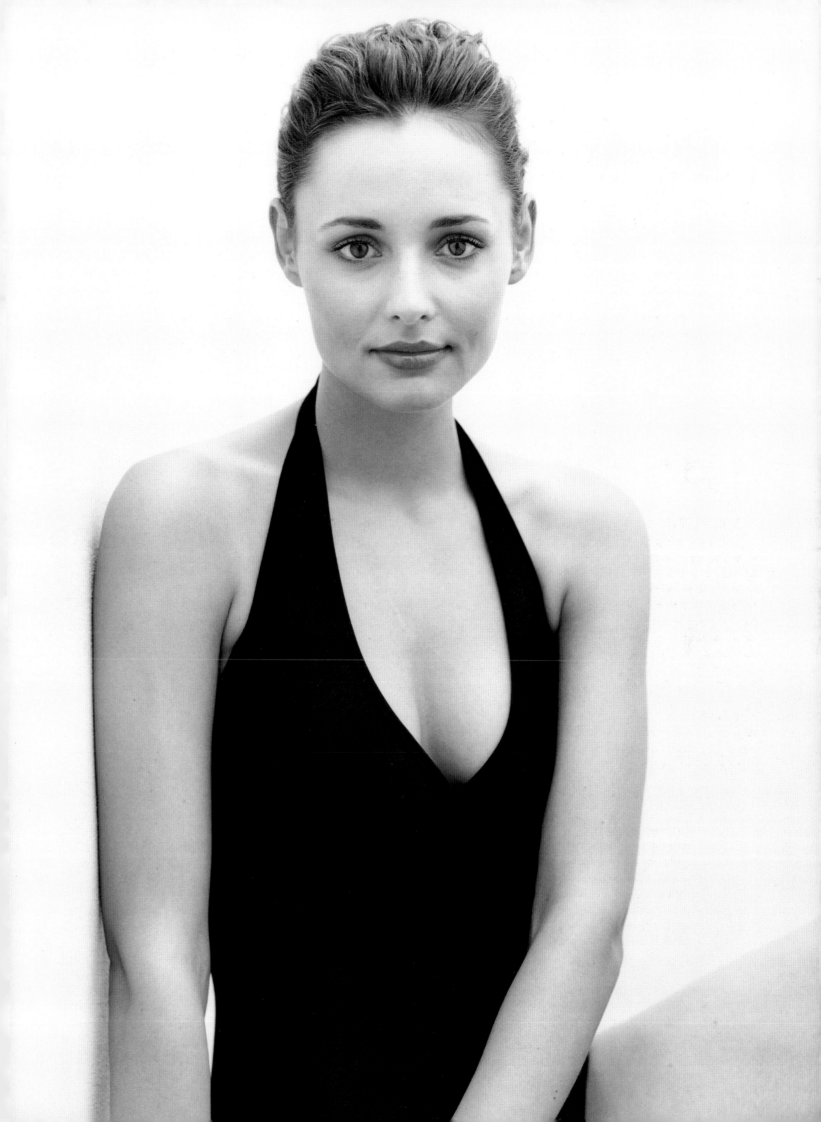

AROMATIC LIVING

FOLLOW THESE STEPS TO INVIGORATE YOUR SENSES

DETOX TREAT

Increase the effectiveness of a detox regime by rubbing the soles of your feet with two drops of juniper oil diluted with 10ml base oil. This will help shift unwanted toxins, as this area relates to the reflex point that regulates kidney function.

BREATHE EASY

Instantly clear your nasal passages if you have a cold, by putting two to three drops of eucalyptus oil on a handkerchief and inhale when required. You can also sprinkle a drop of eucalyptus oil onto your pillow to act as a decongestant at night.

NAIL BOOST

If your nails are prone to breaking, try this blend and store it in a glass bottle: mix 10 drops of lavender, lemon, grapefruit or rosemary oil with one teaspoon of avocado oil. Massage into clean, polish-free nails daily before going to bed.

OVER KILL

If you want to smell different oils to test them, limit your choice to six. Otherwise, you will overload your sense of smell. To improve your sense of smell, have a whiff of a handful of coffee beans in between smelling the different scents.

REVIVING BOOST

For mental and physical exhaustion, mix four drops of lavender oil, three drops each of grapefruit and lemon oil and two drops of sandalwood oil with 25ml almond oil in a glass bottle. Leave to stand for four days before using the blend.

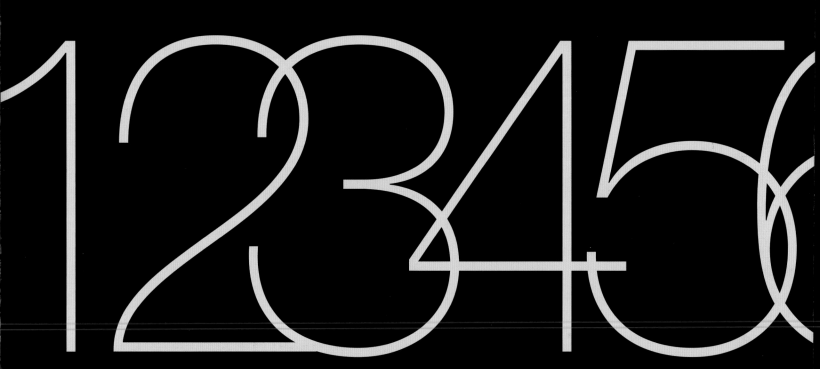

SCENTED APPEAL

Add a couple of drops of lavender oil to the water compartment of your iron and the steam will leave a delicate scent on your clothes. If you have a log fire, add a drop of sandalwood oil to a piece of wood and leave it for 30 minutes before burning.

BURNING ISSUE

To treat minor burns that may occur during cooking or ironing, run the affected area of skin under cold water for at least five minutes. Then gently dab on neat lavender or tea-tree oil to the burn. This will soothe and reduce inflammation.

PAIN RELIEF

If you have a headache, stir one drop each of juniper and fennel essence into 600ml warm water. Soak five cotton-wool pads in the oily solution, wring them out and then place them on your forehead and temples for 10 minutes.

QUALITY CONTROL

Cheap aromatherapy oils are usually chemical copies of natural plant essences and do not have nearly the same medicinal benefits. Opt for reputable brands of essential oils from established stockists or consult an aroma-therapist for advice.

SOOTHE STINGS

Treat wasp or bee stings by applying cider vinegar to the affected area. This will neutralise the poison and help to reduce swelling. Applying a drop of lavender or tea-tree oil mixed with a dessert spoon of vinegar will prevent infection.

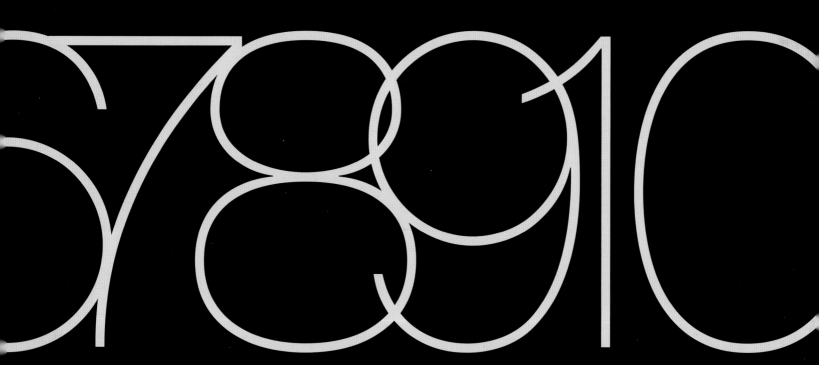

PROBLEM

How should you store essential oils?

Essential oils should be stored in brown glass bottles with air-tight lids, away from light, heat and damp conditions.

What is an effective aromatic treatment for cold sores?

German aromatherapists recommend using melissa oil to treat cold sores. Alternatively, dab on a drop of tea-tree oil using a cotton bud (be careful not to ingest the oil).

What's the best quick-fix for flagging spirits?

Add a drop of eucalyptus oil to a handkerchief and inhale when you're feeling low.

Which essential oils are stress-busters?

Vanilla, nutmeg and orange oils are reputed to calm fraught nerves.

How do you clean an atomiser before adding a new scent?

Rinse the atomiser with vodka, then with water, before filling it with a new scent. This will neutralise the aroma of the previous fragrance.

Which essential oils are aphrodisiacs?
Sandalwood and ylang ylang are the best known aphrodisiac oils.

How does lavender oil help you to sleep?
The aroma stimulates the part of the brain responsible for regulating sleeping patterns.

What's the most effective aromatic wake-up treat?
Add eight drops of your choice of essential oil to your face-cloth or sponge and rub it over your body while in the shower. Breathe in the aromatic steam to revive your senses.

How can you instantly make your surroundings smell good?
Add a couple of drops of your favourite essential oil to a light bulb. The heat of the light will instantly release the aroma.

Should you dab perfume behind your ears?
There are numerous oil glands located behind your ears that can alter the aroma of your fragrance. Dab it onto the inside of your wrists or spray it in your hair instead.

SOLUTION

GLOSSARY

ACIDIC

Solutions that have a pH of less than seven.

ANDROGEN TEST

Determines levels of masculine hormones.

ALKALINE

Substances that have a pH higher than seven.

ALPHA HYDROXY ACIDS (AHAs)

Also known as fruit acids, these substances break down the intercellular glue that adheres dead cells to the face and body.

ALLERGEN

A substance that causes an allergic reaction.

AMINO ACIDS

Molecules that are linked together to form proteins. They are the main constituents of skin and hair.

BASAL CELLS

Cells found in the germination layer of the epidermis.

BASE OIL

(Also called carrier oil.) Inert vegetable or mineral oils used in aromatherapy to blend with essential oils. These oils do not alter the properties of essential oils, instead, they reduce the concentration of essential oils to make aromatherapy blends safer. Jojoba, sweet almond, avocado and wheatgerm are commonly used as base oils.

COLLAGEN

The fibrous substance found in the dermis that gives skin its support, elasticity, strength, and suppleness.

CORTEX

The inner layer of hair. Made of fibre-like cells, the cortex gives hair its strength and elasticity. It also houses the colour pigments that determine natural hair colour.

CUTICLES

The outer layer of hair that is structured with tiny, overlapping scales. When these scales lie flat, light is reflected evenly by the hair's surface, making locks appear healthy and shiny. If cuticles are damaged by over-zealous shampooing, chemical processing or neglect, they won't sit properly and the hair will look dull, lifeless and brittle.

DERMIS

The tough layer of skin below the epidermis containing collagen and elastin. The dermis houses the sebaceous glands, blood vessels, hair follicles, sweat glands and nerve endings – the skin's sensory receptors.

EPIDERMIS

The outer layer of the skin, which protects the body from external environmental aggressors, such

as ultraviolet rays and pollution. The epidermis is made up of both living and dead skin cells.

ELASTIN

The fibres that constitute most of the elastic tissue in the body and the skin. These fibres break down with age, causing skin to sag.

ENZYMES

Proteins formed in cells that act as catalysts in biochemical reactions.

FREE RADICALS

Rogue molecules that have a degenerative effect on the body and accelerate the ageing process.

HOLISTIC

A philosophy or approach that encompasses total well-being. The holistic approach treats a person as a whole entity, rather than isolating a problem or pain. It focuses on addressing imbalances within the body that result in illness.

KERATIN

Strands of protein found in the skin, hair and nails.

LYMPHATIC SYSTEM

Complex internal waste disposal system. Lymph, a clear fluid, circulates through the body transporting waste materials. This waste is disposed of

at lymphatic glands (or nodes) – special ducts in different regions of the body, such as under the arms or behind the knees.

MEDULLA

The core that runs through the middle of each hair shaft. The medulla is believed to carry nutrients and other substances to the cortex and cuticles.

MELANIN

The skin's natural colour pigment. The colour of skin is determined by the activity of melanin-producing cells, called melanocytes. Dark skins contain a high concentration of melanin and very active melanocytes, while fair skins have partially coloured melanin granules. In addition, melanin is the body's natural sun defence mechanism. During sun exposure, the body produces more melanin to protect the skin. This activity temporarily darkens the skin, creating a suntan.

METABOLISM

The combination of chemical processes within the body, such as the conversion of food into energy, the excretion of waste, and the regulation of growth. These activities slow down with age.

ORBITAL BONE

The small bone located directly under the eye.

PABA

A chemical sunscreen used in sun-protection products.

PH

A scale that determines whether a substance is acid or alkaline. The pH scale ranges from 0 to 14. The range between 0 and 7 is acidic and between 7 and 14 is alkaline, while 7 is neutral. The natural pH of skin and hair is slightly acidic. Cosmetic preparations are adjusted to suit this.

RETIN-A

(Also called retinoic acid.) A derivative of retinol (vitamin A), initially developed as a treatment for acne. It is now used as an anti-ageing treatment to help diminish fine lines and wrinkles.

SEBACEOUS GLANDS

The network of glands that produce sebum.

SEBUM

Oily substance that acts as a natural lubricant to hydrate and protect skin and hair.

STRATUM CORNEUM

The outermost layer of the epidermis. Skin cells travel from the lower levels of the skin to the epidermis. When they arrive at the strateum corneum, they are dead and eventually shed. This cycle takes approximately 28 days in healthy skins, but slows down with age.

INDEX